# GET YOUR BACK BACK

# GET
# YOUR BACK
# BACK

## Break Free from Back Pain—
## No Surgery, No Meds, No Nonsense!

### ALISTAIR McKENZIE

IZZARD INK
PUBLISHING®

IZZARD INK PUBLISHING
www.izzardink.com

Library of Congress Cataloging-in-Publication Data

Names: McKenzie, Alistair (Alistair Fergus) author
Title: Get your back back / Alistair McKenzie.
Description: First edition. | [Salt Lake City] : Izzard Ink Publishing,
    [2025] | Includes bibliographical references.
Identifiers: LCCN 2025029892 (print) | LCCN 2025029893 (ebook) | ISBN
    9781642281316 hardback | ISBN 9781642281309 paperback | ISBN
    9781642281293 ebook | ISBN 9781642281323 ebook
Subjects: LCSH: Backache—Treatment
Classification: LCC RD771.B217 M427 2025 (print) | LCC RD771.B217 (ebook)
LC record available at https://lccn.loc.gov/2025029892
LC ebook record available at https://lccn.loc.gov/2025029893

*Designed by Daniel Lagin*
Cover Design by Andrea Ho
Cover Images by Andrea Ho
Interior Drawings by Mika McMillan lupenzart@gmail.com

First Edition
Contact the author at www.corecraft.co.nz
eBook ISBN: 978-1-64228-129-3
Paperback ISBN: 978-1-64228-130-9
Hardback ISBN: 978-1-64228-131-6
Audiobook ISBN: 978-1-64228-132-3

*For Nola*

# CONTENTS

# INTRODUCTION

*"Our body is like a dog waiting for its master, the brain,
to throw it a stick. Once comfortable with this awareness,
we can relax in the knowledge that every thought matters."*

**—ALISTAIR MCKENZIE**

Over the past twenty-five years working in the massage industry, I have found it instrumental to bridge the practical insights of manual therapy with the emotional aspects of healing. *Get Your Back Back* offers an effective approach to understanding and treating body pain based on what I have learned and experienced from my own pain journey and from working with clients. Within these pages, I reveal what generates the common body pains many of us endure and explain how *elevated stress levels* are the most significant factor that sets this pain in motion. This is why managing stress (emotional) and integrating supportive and restorative body movements (physical) make such a balanced pair. Balance is such an important word in regaining healthy physical and emotional vitality. Anything done to the extreme will always lead to poor outcomes. Escalating life pressures increase body tension to the point where body failures are triggered. Steadily accumulating muscle tension pressurizes blood vessels and nerves, which then radiate pain and dysfunction to remote sites of the body. For example, a sore calf muscle is usually caused by spinal nerve pressure one-third of the way up the back of the ribcage. Aching shoulders are a symptom of active pressure points on the front of the neck, brought on by dysfunctional breathing techniques. These dull, throbbing aches are easily misdiagnosed as rotator cuff injuries. Back pains and sciatica are usually stress-related.

My goal is to offer you the option of disconnecting from the current tsunami of misinformation surrounding ill health. We could collectively save an enormous amount of time, money, and valuable resources by shifting our focus to the true origin of most of our "dis-eases," which are stress-related body tensions. This requires a major shift into embracing hands-on diagnosis. My techniques have helped many to better understand and resolve their body pains. I hope it can also help you find healing as you look deeper for the root causes and stop treating the symptoms in isolation. This book will shed light on some popular health misconceptions and lead you to begin asking, "Why does it *really* hurt there?"

## MY STORY

Looking back over family photos, my smile was always ear to ear. People probably thought I was really happy, but my grin was driven by anxiety, similar to that of monkeys in a study of fear responses in primates.[1] As a child, I was afraid of my mother and terrified of my father. Both were very clever and hardworking people, and it seemed to me that there was nothing they could not do on their 200-acre hobby farm. My siblings and I always had shelter and plenty of food, but I had no feeling of safety or recognition. The terms of our child labor were very simple. It was our job to *help* with whatever needed doing on the day. There was never any consultation or discussion about it. My mother would simply say, "I think your father needs a hand with . . ." (whatever it was she saw him head off to do). I'm not even sure they ever discussed the rules and structure of the family unit with one another. How long any of us might be needed for any one of these tasks would come down to how long it took. Jobs like weeding the one acre of the vegetable garden, plucking and gutting poultry, processing vegetables, scraping the hair off scalded pigs, herding animals, picking up stones, and building new fences after removing the old ones are just a few of the regular farm tasks we did. These jobs just had to be done. The list seemed never-ending and would cycle around to repeat every year. The gap between the six of us children and consultation widened further at the end of each job as we simply wandered off when we guessed that what we had been needed for was complete. I do remember being fascinated by the anatomy of the slaughtered birds and animals. Plucking and gutting them always turned into dissection as I delved into their inner workings. I took a lot longer than I should have down in the creek bed as the eels, drawn in by the watery smell of blood, came in for their share. I was able to cut open the heart and study its valves, held by tiny strands of stringy tissue. I pulled the skin off the liver and wondered at its curiously dark, grainy texture, then sliced the kidneys open and followed the blood vessels as they disappeared into the tissue. There was not a single component that escaped my curiosity. One of the most memorable was holding a pig's lungs under a running water tap and expanding them out to around four times their resting size.

An incessant worrier, my mother's communication style was very much "her way or the highway." I know she wanted to treat me warmly, but her goodnight hugs felt brittle and always ended with her hands on my shoulders, pushing me away, a bit like an exclamation mark at the end of a sentence. This squeeze was always followed by, "Give your father a kiss." I always dreaded this, hoping he had no reason to lash out as I bent forward and kissed him on his motionless five-o'clock shadowed cheek. As was the case in most homes in the fifties and sixties, my mother did all of the housework and my father was the breadwinner. My father was a smoldering volcano. He was well balanced with enormous chips on both of his shoulders and seemed to be perpetually pissed off. He worked the land every weekend and after 3:30 every working day, only coming into the house at mealtimes, or to sleep.

For the most part, I was able to avoid my father until my fifth birthday. From that day until I was twelve, I had to be with him Monday through Friday from nine o'clock until three o'clock. There I sat, frozen in fear, in a tiny school chair at a wee lift-top school desk with a ceramic inkwell in the top right-hand corner. It turned out that I was soon to learn why we use the term "I was shitting myself." A man whom I hardly knew was our only teacher. Kokiri school, ten miles from the next town, stood alone on a terrace above the winter fog. Bathed in sunshine, its location was the envy of the valley residents. This West Coast town of six houses, nicknamed "Foggy Bottom," had more wet days than sunshine and a daily winter fog that hung over the houses, sometimes until one o'clock in the afternoon. This was a sole-charge school with a roll of about eighteen children. On that first day, too scared to ask him if I could use the toilet, I soiled my pants, and once the smell reached his nostrils, I was sent back down the half-mile gravel road to our home. Witnessing my father lifting his dogs off the ground by their collar and beating them over and over with a stick had already galvanized my fear of him. Especially that one time when I noticed the dog, that had received a beating the day before, was no longer in its kennel. I still remember as if it were yesterday, his huge hand clamped across the back of my neck, forcing my face into the page of my school workbook.

I learned very early on to *become invisible* and *keep my head down.* I did not see any of my older brothers' beatings until years later, but I had heard them. One time my mother let out a shriek from the kitchen, threw the sliding door open, and yelled, "Put him down!" I have no recollection of what I had done wrong, but my father had grabbed me

by the hair, lifted me off the ground, and was shaking me. Thank God
he dropped me and I was able to run out of the room. Another incident
I experienced turned my fear of my father into terror. I was supposed
to be holding onto the pipe that ran along the side of the swimming
pool and was kicking my feet with my face in the water while turning
my head to the side to take a breath. Having my face in the water
always made me feel panicky, and I couldn't do it. So he grabbed my
head, pushed my face into the water, and held it there. Something happens deep inside when the one person who is meant to keep you safe
shows you that he can threaten your existence! In that moment, his
power over me was complete. Corporal punishment was considered
acceptable in the sixties, but surely there must have been rules for
that! Yet because he ran the school singlehandedly, my father had
total control. This meant that in cases of punishment, he was judge,
jury, and executioner all rolled into one. And there I stood with my
arm held out, guilty. He always kept the leather straps in full view. One
was always rolled up on the top of his school desk, and another was
on display in the kitchen at home. The full force of this school strap
swung down from where it rested over his shoulder. Not just onto my
hand but over my whole lower arm. The pain was instant and searing.
I still remember that burning red glow that stayed for hours. His physical dominance over me was complete but more damaging I think was
his psychological dominance. Knowing protest was futile and the
absence of anyone safe to tell created a void full of unresolved feelings.

One evening when I was eleven, I had no idea he was waiting on
the other side of the sliding door to the kitchen until his fist landed
squarely on my face. Running from the house and needing to feel safe,
I hid in the dog kennel behind one of the farm dogs. My sister found
me hours later and had brought me a mutton chop from the tea table.
Knowing that my cover was blown, I crept over the handmade swing
bridge to the shearing shed and hid underneath, crouching above the
layer of sheep shit that covered the ground. A couple of hours later I
was in my bed, eyes wide open, barely breathing. My fear of the dark

had driven me back into the house where I had crept past that closed kitchen door into my bedroom. Because it was the weekend, I knew if I was late for breakfast, my father would already be outside. My mother said he thought I had stolen his cigarettes. I had not. Nothing more was ever said.

Throughout my early adult years, I struggled with my inability to communicate. My adult relationships collapsed through my lack of understanding of how healthy relationships function at that point. Adding to my life's pressure, I was on the edge of being made redundant for eight years. Eventually, I was laid off and began exploring my next career path: massage therapy. Partway through the year, one of my tutors at the college, Eddie Guzy, handed me a brochure. It was an advertisement for a men's retreat organized by a nonprofit called Men's Trust. Attending that weekend course turned into a watershed for me. There were exercises designed to get us running around and making noise to stir us up, followed by seated silence. The thirty of us sat in a large circle, listened to a presentation by the instructor, and began to tell our stories. One man held the talking stick and spoke while the rest listened. Feedback was only ever offered, and the key ingredients to the group were safety, nonviolence (both verbal and physical), and total confidentiality. Up to that point, I had no idea what it meant to be a man. I foolishly thought that men all had to be the same. Listening to their stories, I discovered each man was a unique individual. I realized that in order to become the man that I was searching to be was false. All I ever needed to be was myself.

Following the introductory event, I attended a number of others, all at isolated locations. Each of these provided their own growth opportunities, none less than a men's and boys' trip to Westland's Paparoa National Park. A Department of Conservation ranger started the retreat with a safety briefing. He said that flood was a major risk in these steep-sided valleys and we were to take no risks. A particularly loud member of the group decided to take it upon himself to lead the boys up a river canyon in spite of a storm warning announced for later that day. The only one with local knowledge, I suggested to him that I would call emergency services if they were not back at the car park by 3 o'clock, to which he nonchalantly agreed.

Soon after their departure, the stream morphed into a raging river, carrying debris out to sea. I was hoping no boys' bodies were among those floating tree trunks. The 3 o'clock deadline came and went, and there was no sign of the group. I went back to base camp told the retreat leader what was happening, and he said to wait, so I returned to the track car park and waited. Forty-five minutes later, the group arrived soaking wet, laughing and joking. They had been playing in the floodwaters along the side of the valley. I was incredibly angry but of course unable to express how I felt. Later that night I was trying to sleep but my body would not let me. My belly was churning, I felt hot, and I was sweating. Hearing the men laughing and joking in the lounge made me even more unsettled. I had read the book *Feel the Fear and Do It Anyway* by Susan Jeffers,[2] so I leapt out of bed and, with my heart pounding, went downstairs. I told the group that I thought this man had acted irresponsibly and had risked the lives of other people's children against the clear instructions given to us by the park ranger. His total disregard for the agreement we had made was evident. Following a discussion in the group, the man apologized to me. I went back to bed. My tummy had settled, my heart rate returned to normal, and I slept soundly right through the night. I was finally learning how to communicate in a safe and direct way, which brought an inevitable end to my second marriage. The other valuable lesson I learned was the direct connection between stressful situations and our body. I learned that we *can* have an actual fire in our belly. It gets hot and actually hurts. We can get the runs, get sweaty, and lie awake with an increased heart rate. In fact, our whole-body chemistry changes with stress and is driven by our thoughts. The legacy of my less-than-perfect childhood had me holding lower body tension, which eventually squeezed a bubble out the side of one of the discs in the base of my back. That disc protrusion compressed the sciatic nerve, sending agonizing pain all the way to my heel.

## MY PAIN EXPERIENCE

I share my pain experience so that you can see that not only do I know what it's like to live with chronic pain but to let you know I have been partway down the medical route, that for a lot of patients ends at the pain management clinic. My daily pain management routine began early. After yet another restless night where it was impossible to get comfortable, I reached out for the side of the mattress with one hand, being *very* careful not to move my torso, and dragged myself to the side of the bed. I knew that if I tried to turn over or sit up, my pain levels would rocket to an unbearable ten out of ten. In what is best described as a controlled fall, I eased my feet gingerly onto the floor, legs outstretched. Resting for a while on my knees for a few deep breaths, the difficult work of standing up began. This was the most painful part, and I dreaded it every morning. Knowing full well that my left leg was the more comfortable option, I gingerly brought it forward at a controlled rate so as not to send a shock wave down my other leg. Ever so slowly, I got vertical with the help of a large bedside cabinet and the side of the mattress for support. Throughout this process of going from kneeling to standing, there were the usual oohs and aahs, with more than a few profanities mixed in. Walking was nearly as dramatic.

I had one good leg and one weak leg that kept me in constant pain. Knowing it could go out from under me at any time, I hobbled down the hallway. My daily agonizing ritual then took me to the freezer, where I selected an ice pack, wrapped it in a small towel, and placed it under the belt of my dressing gown in the center of my lower back. I learned early on that although heat packs felt really comforting, the chill of the ice pack was much more effective at dulling my pain. About twenty minutes later, I headed off to the freezer again to replace the

warmed ice pack for another frozen one. Sitting also had to be carefully choreographed. Anything of normal height was way too low, so I
resorted to perching on the edge of the sofa arms. Thank goodness my
vehicle wasn't the kind I had to step down into because I don't think I
could have done it. My trusty "truck" was a Nissan Navara double cab,
so it was a good height, but even that took an age to get inside. With
such a tight back, my neck couldn't flex far enough forward to get
under the roof support! My head had to go in first, carefully followed
by the rest of my body in a sideways leaning roll. I know this is all
starting to sound ridiculous, but I really had no other option. I was
stuck with this pain (or so I thought), and medication was struggling
to put a dent in providing any lasting relief. I could not drive far without stopping to tip the seat back as far as it could go. In this position,
I could push myself back, then, with my feet firmly planted on the
floor, I'd lift my bottom off the seat and hold it up for a minute or two,
forcing the pain that I called "the rats" to take a break from chewing
on the back of my leg! Looking back, I'm not really sure how I was able
to stand long enough to work at all, but I did find a way (standing on
mostly one leg!).

Through the medical system I was offered cortisone injections
and the possibility of surgery. The orthopedic specialist informed me
that I would be referred to the pain management clinic if the procedure was not successful. Not satisfied with the odds of being pain-free
at the end of that process I hobbled away to continue my search for
another solution. When I finally steered my life in a different direction
and connected with Dr. Joe Brownlee, everything shifted, including
my painful condition. Following my own recovery, I delved into the
mystery of why *most people* suffer from body pain and some degree of
skeletal imbalance. Why is pain the norm instead of the exception? I
will address these concerns and my discoveries throughout this book.

Most of the activities offered in here are specifically designed to
be incorporated seamlessly into your day. The micro improvements
introduced throughout the chapters are repeated in Chapter 19,

Repairs and Maintenance, in order to easily access them again. The Common Language statements at the beginning of each chapter are samplings of the mind-body connections we subconsciously make conversationally. We unknowingly describe the location of the pain/issue with this negative talk, and in some cases, we even identify the type and level of the upset, tension, and "dis-ease." This *under-the-radar* language is initiated by our reactions to everyday situations. The Quick Fixes that follow contain the essence of each chapter, which you may find useful for revision. In some of these, I have added positive changes that you may adopt. A great deal of my learning came from witnessing the individual experiences of my clients. As you read on, you will come across their stories, and I hope you can relate to some. I have collectively named my clients either Mary or Peter in the interest of anonymity.

# CHAPTER 1

# OUT OF WHACK

## COMMON LANGUAGE

*"She is bitter and twisted."*
*"I wouldn't buy a thing from him. He is crooked."*
*"Keeps me on the straight and narrow."*

## QUICK FIX

The core foundation of our body is the pelvis, and it can get twisted (or "out of whack") through physical injury or overexposure to psychological stress. This foundational distortion angulates all of the body's structures, producing chronic pain, movement restrictions, and individual component failures. These pelvic distortional body pains and dysfunctions are treatable.

Our pelvis is recognized by many in the medical community as a solid unit, and for the duration of my therapeutic massage training, I also believed this to be true. My classmates and I studied human anatomy and physiology, learned how to locate and restore muscle function, and became skilled in balancing tilted pelvises. We were taught that the remedy for a client's off-center posture was to identify, massage, and stretch the offending *muscles*, not the *structure*. Once put into practice though, this method did not prove to be reliable. During my training, I listened to the instructors, treating the muscles, which yielded varying results, but I never succeeded in fully correcting any-one's posture. Sometimes the client would feel a lot better after the massage, but most of the time I could tell that they were only margin-ally better, if that. When I asked, "How do you feel now?" they would automatically answer, "Really good. Thank you." Or they'd politely say, "Much better." I got the feeling some of them were simply glad I had stopped digging my thumbs into their muscles. But something bigger was concerning me at the beginning of my career, and I was deter-mined to stay awake and aware for how I could better serve my clients.

It was while treating the neck of a new client for the first time that my breakthrough began. I had been uncomfortable with the fact that the treatment massages I was delivering seemed relatively ineffective. Seeing the same person over and over offered little more than tempo-rary pain relief. While I fully endorse and encourage regular mainte-nance massage sessions as a necessary part of a well-balanced self-care regime, I had been seeing the same people repeatedly for what was, in most cases, relatively serious levels of musculoskeletal dysfunction. I was frustrated in knowing that there must be some-thing more effective that could be done, so I continued pushing the envelope by enrolling in advanced training classes and reading all I could on the matter. Over the next few years, I pioneered my own technique: "Core Craft Manual Therapy." The word *core* relates to the weakened central area (midline) of our bodies where we hold our feel-ings. This part of ourselves that we hide away from the world to keep ourselves *safe* is more often than not the origin of our *physical* dys-function. I included the word *craft* because of the individual nature of the work. As I continued to develop and fine-tune my new method, I noticed the same clients I had been seeing for chronic pain began to steadily improve. With far more positive outcomes becoming the new norm, my technique was abuzz throughout the community. My regu-lars needed less pain management, so my business shifted away from a caged-bird system into something that resembled a catch-and-release method. My clients began referring friends and family members. One of these new clients delivered what turned out to be my lightbulb opportunity within their first few minutes of treatment.

"Oh my God!" she began excitedly. "You work in a very similar way to Dr. Joe Brownlee. He is desperately seeking someone to pass his skills on to. I can give you his number if you like."

Curious, I gave him a call that same morning. Not only did I want to enhance my skill level, I hoped Dr. Brownlee could finally be the one to fix my back! After all, I needed help with my pain much like my clients! Dr. Brownlee answered his phone while on the golf course mid-game and sounded genuinely overjoyed by my request to meet with him. He had a warm personality and explained his work history: He began in agricultural contracting and farming, then went on to medical university and became a general practitioner. More recently, he had become a practitioner of musculoskeletal therapy, obtaining his diploma at age sixty-five. It turned out that Dr. Joe (as I came to call him) had been trained in a unique form of bodywork technique by Karl Levett from Czechoslovakia. He followed up on my request for advanced training by inviting me into his clinic for two-hour sessions every Monday morning. This he did in the hope that I might "finally be the one to continue his legacy." He used the word *finally* because all of those who had trained under him so far had "not had it in their hands." Those words instantly took me back to a time years ago when I was doing a bit of massage and bodywork on a few of my friends for a hobby. They suggested I give up my day job and do bodywork for a living. The reason? "Because you've got good hands."

Dr. Joe exuded quiet confidence with his full head of carefully combed white hair and spotless medical coat. His knowing smile seemed to fill the room. I didn't find out until much later that having been irreplaceable at the Papanui Musculoskeletal Clinic, he had been called back from retirement twice already. He was a living legend to many of his patients, some of whom later relayed stories of patients going into his clinic on crutches and walking out with the crutches under their arms.

Dr. Joe said, "Before I begin, you have to promise me two things. This work is unique and very important. You have to write the book I never did and then pass on this *hands-on method* I am about to teach you to someone else before you die."

Knowing that I had already amassed a stack of notes containing my own clinical findings and eager to learn more, I swiftly promised to do both. I had no way of knowing at that early stage that it would take a full three years until that the baton would finally be passed to me. Following a brief explanation to his first patient of the day as to why I was there, and after gaining their approval to continue, he began. In the moments that followed, I understood his use of the term *hands-on method* as he gently but firmly sandwiched my hands between the exposed skin of his patient and his own hands. Using my thumb as a tool and my fingers as the guides, he swiftly located where his patient's tissues had become *stuck*. I knew in an instant that my own treatment method would never be the same again. I also knew, without a doubt, that I would (proudly and with great honor) write his book. I watched attentively as Dr. Joe demonstrated how to check his patient's leg lengths both while lying down and while sitting up.

Moments after asking his patient to turn over and lie face down on his treatment table, I had my eureka moment. While hooking the fingers of my right hand under his patient's right side and pressing my left hand onto the base of their spine, Dr. Joe said the magic words as casually as if asking if I would prefer a cup of tea or coffee at ten o'clock: "*We are now realigning the pelvic joints.*" You could have knocked me over with a feather. Somehow I intuitively knew it must be possible to naturally release the body. But up to that moment, I had never been able to figure out what the "it" factor was. Finally, my answer had come. This was my holy grail moment.

Dr. Joe's words had confirmed that the pelvis wasn't a solid unit at all. The three main bones that form our pelvis (the sacrum and two iliums) can become twisted and jammed, causing negative consequences for the whole body. And the best part? Pelvic misalignment is treatable!

## "OUT OF WHACK" CHECK

People have described their painfully bent bodies to me in lots of ways, but one of the most common and the one that has stuck is when they say, *"I feel out of whack."* To find whether or not you are out of whack, do the following:

*Lie flat on the floor and have a friend look at the wee bumps on your inner ankles. Do not check by looking at the toes because they can move independently, giving a false reading. Are your ankle bumps directly opposite? If the answer is no, this is great news for you because you probably have an* **apparent leg length difference***, which may cause any of a very long list of body symptoms. Next move up to sitting with your legs still lying flat. In this position your friend will more than likely notice that your leg lengths almost equalize. (In the seated position the upper leg bone femoral heads are raised and lowered instead of being extended and retracted.)*

## "APPARENT" LEG LENGTH DIFFERENCE

I say *apparent* length difference because, in my twenty-five years of practice, I have seen only *two* clients with one leg actually shorter than the other. If you are out of whack, your pelvis will have twisted and locked, pulling one leg toward you and pushing the other slightly farther away. In this state, you cannot sit or stand straight or have a pain-free, fully functional body. Most people I see through my clinic who are out of whack make a full recovery once successfully realigned. If you are out of whack, it will probably be the right leg that *seems*

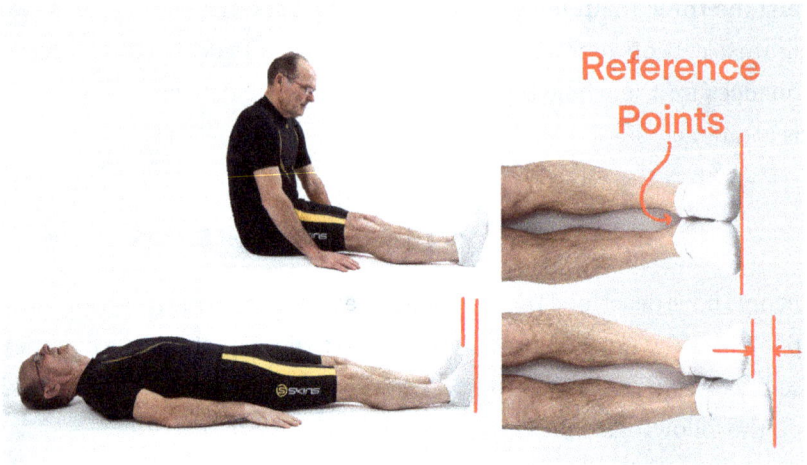

*shorter.* In my experience, only 5 percent of people who are carrying this imbalance are shortened on the left side.

## SELF CHECK

*If there is no one around to do the check for you, sit with your left foot on your right knee, then slide your left foot along your thigh toward your tummy. Remembering how far your foot slid along, change over, doing the*

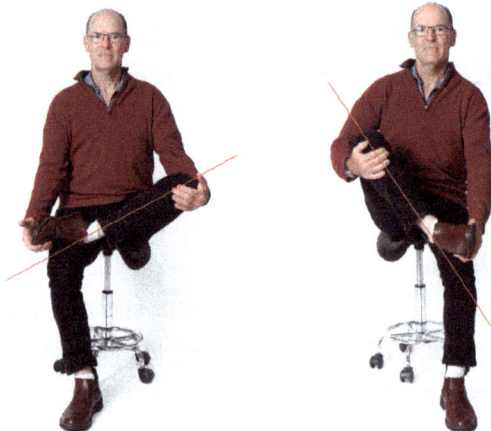

*same test on the other side. If one foot doesn't slide as far along, or one of*
*your held knees raises higher, chances are good you are out of whack.*
*(This test is not something that can easily be measured, but any tension*
*or leg height difference between the two sides will be obvious.)*

## THE PELVIC JOINTS

The picture below shows what your pelvis, lower back, and hips look like
when viewed from the front. You have three joints in your pelvis, but
you can only ever feel the joint at the front (pubic symphysis). The other
two (sacroiliac joints) are concealed at the base of your spine. These
three are not like any others in your body because they are not shiny
and don't slide one bone over the other. They are connected by a tough,
fibrous material that allows your tiny, internalized tail at the bottom
end of your sacrum to wag from side to side a few millimeters with
every step. Once forced past the end of their natural travel, they get
jammed, stopping any tail wagging and causing your back to go "out."

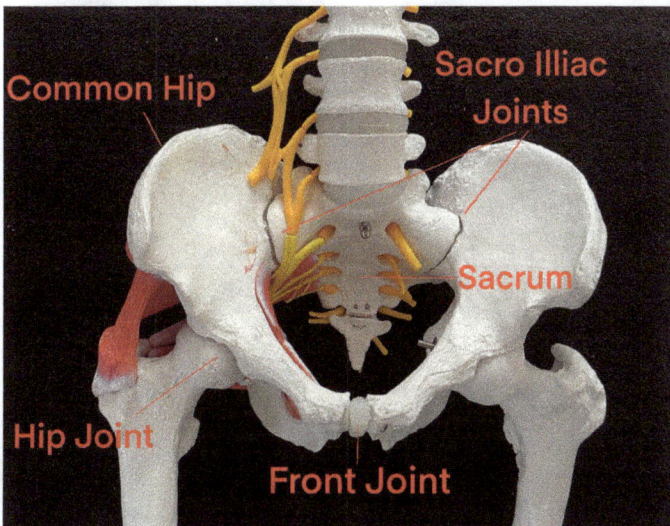

## SO WHERE IS "OUT"?

If the muscles holding the pelvis in place are stronger on one side, the *whole pelvis* tends to tilt to the weakened side. In this case, the relationship between the pelvic bones does not change. Closer inspection of the photo again demonstrates this. You can see that although the spine is vertical, the pelvis is lower on the left and higher on the right. The key to seeing that there is no rotation of the joints is the bottom tip of the sacrum still lining up with the front joint. There is a fairly simple fix for this *tilt* that only requires deep-tissue massage to release any holding on the shortened side and strengthening of the muscles on the weakened side.

The first of these next two images shows the pelvic bones and joints in correct functional alignment. The sacrum is vertical, and the joint at the front is level. The second image shows how pelvic rotation negatively affects all of the components. The right side of the pelvis has rotated backward, and the left has rotated forward. This has stretched the pubic symphysis joint at the front up on the right

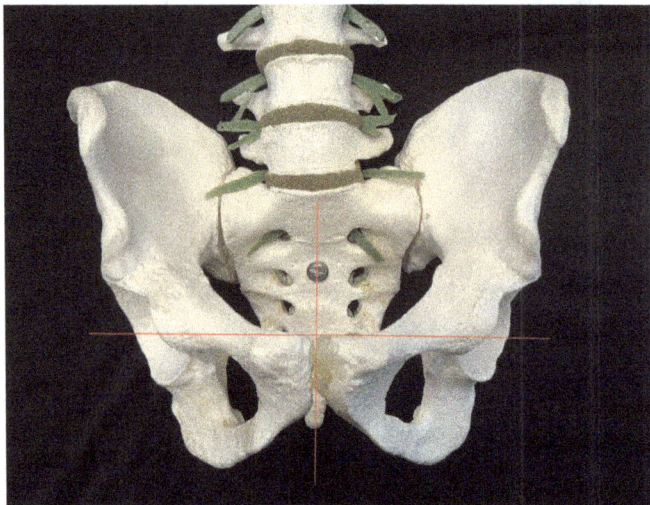

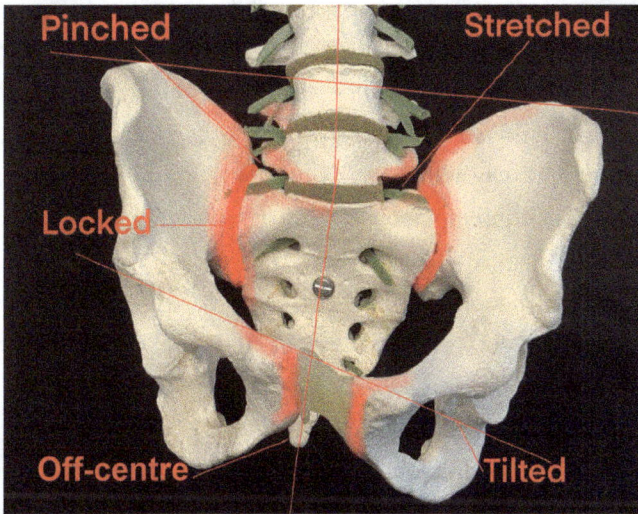

and down on the left. The sacrum has been pulled off-center, crushing one side of the lower spine and overstretching the other side. Joint inflammation is highlighted in red.

In a body that is out of whack, the hip bones rotate in opposite directions, twisting and jamming the sacrum off-center. This seemingly insignificant sacral bone has a crucial role to play in our bodies as it forms our foundations. The lower body hangs from your pelvis, and the upper body rests down onto it. To help put this imagery into perspective, we all know the foundation under a building has to be level. If any foundation has slumped on one corner, all of the doors and windows get stuck and will not function (open/close) properly. But it's not because there is anything wrong with any of them. The fault lies entirely with the base of the building. A builder could go around and ease all of those door and window frames, but leveling the foundations will fix them all at once. Our bodies don't have doors and windows; what gets stuck is all of our moving parts, such as our neck, shoulders, back, knees, and the list goes on throughout the body.

MARY (All my female clients will be referred to as Mary in this book, but their stories all differ, just as we all differ as individuals.)

*I see Mary about twice yearly for a bit of neck and shoulder stiffness and a painfully swollen left knee (Mary's doors and windows). Knowing that her knee is symptomatic of her crooked foundations, I never touch it. With her sacrum rebalanced, the knee stops hurting and the swelling goes away within a few days. The neck and shoulder only ever need a bit of gentle mobilizing once her foundations are successfully rebalanced.*

I often find people who begin treatment with a 1.5 or even 2.5 centimeter pelvic distortion. *(The term "pelvic distortion" refers to the three bones that form the pelvis, oppositely rotating in relation to one another, twisting and locking the sacrum away from horizontal.)* I can assure you that this foundational shift affecting everything in your body is not an exaggeration. Once the base of your spine tilts to the side, *all* of your spinal bones and the surrounding muscles must adjust to compensate. This means that everything that was balancing now has to be held, and all of the holding needs to be constantly adjusted to

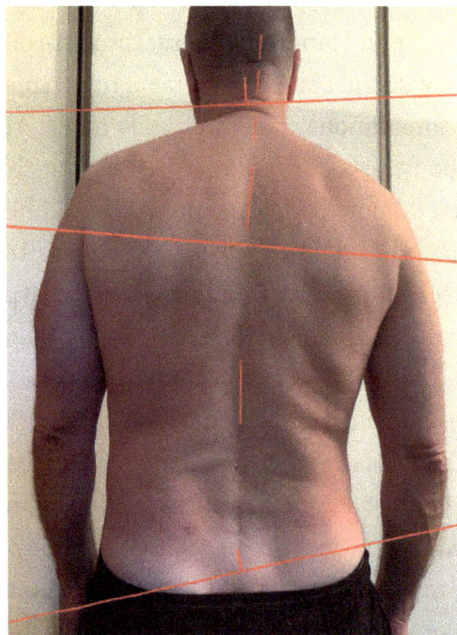

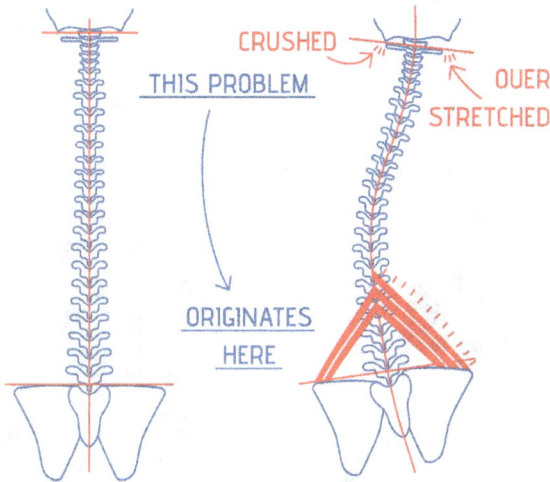

manage the abnormal twisting and turning. Your subconscious *normal* muscle settings need to be reprogrammed into the *new normal* with every muscle operating longer or shorter depending on their positioning. The vertebral misalignment and muscular tension required to manage this distortion reduces overall spinal mobility to 50 percent of what is accepted as normal. The top vertebra, which allows the head to swivel and nod, has another valuable function: balance. This *body-spirit level* needs to be totally free to move in any direction, allowing its imaginary bubble to return to resting in the middle. This essential top bone echoes any sideways tilting at the base of the spine. If you find that you are out of whack and want to know if it has spread all the way to the top of your spine, just look over each shoulder. See if one side goes farther. *Peter pictured on previous page, has a pelvic rotation of 2.5 centimeters. His body's S-bended response is obvious.*

Whereas a balanced body automatically returns to balance, a body that is out of whack always returns to imbalance. Living out of whack makes it impossible for you to get comfortable sitting, lying down, or standing straight, as your body literally forces you crookedly "onto the back foot." It is way more than just important to have your sacrum free-floating and able to come to rest, level in the center.

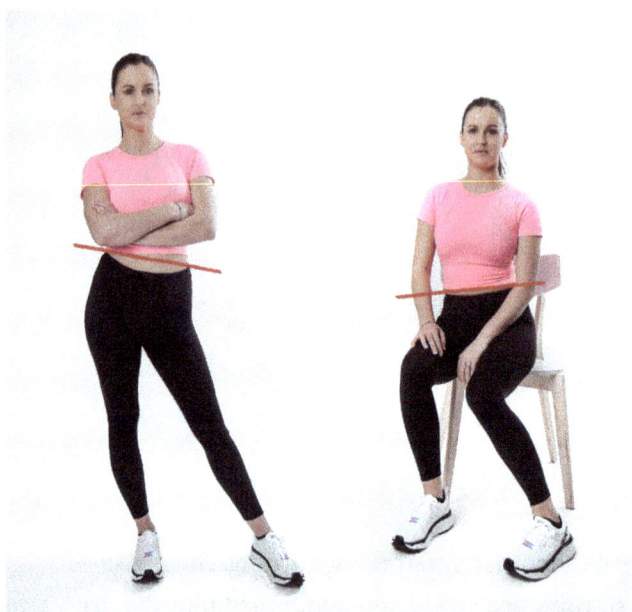

It is crucial (see Chapter 19, Repairs and Maintenance for remedial self-treatments).

## THREE POSSIBLE CAUSES
## OF PELVIC DISTORTION

### 1. Repetitive Asymmetrical Exercise

Anyone doing repetitive weight bearing exercise runs the risk of becoming unbalanced themselves. Exercise builds body strength and fitness, and if this is done often enough in one direction, one side becomes much stronger, which inevitably shifts the skeleton off-center. A full recovery is possible only once the muscles are equalized. This can be difficult to achieve if doing something like shoveling, stacking timber, or playing professional golf. We all have a favorite "go to" side (right or left), which feels a lot more coordinated and comfortable to use. If you are a golfer, it's worth buying a club for your opposite swing and whacking a few to your uncoordinated side off the practice range each time you go out. With manual labor like shoveling or stacking wood, force yourself to keep changing sides at regular intervals. It feels counterintuitive at first, yet balancing your whole self in this way will eventually feel natural.

## 2. Physical Trauma

The joints of the pelvis are really tough and don't move far, but with enough force from a sudden impact, they can be shifted. It takes quite a hit to get them to move, but there is no mistaking once it happens. It's the kind of violent impact that leaves you stunned. And even though you don't quite know what happened, there is no doubt that something major has just gone wrong. Falling onto your butt will do it. The origin may be snowboarding, ice skating, mountain biking, even a long-forgotten jungle-gym accident or a school chair pulled out from under you when you were sitting down. Car accidents are another common cause. Having the pelvis and only one shoulder held firmly by lap and diagonal seat belts throws the unrestrained side of the upper body forward, violently rotating the spine, which tears the immobilized pelvic joints off-center. Childbirth trauma can misalign the pelvis of the baby and or mother. Both could be routinely checked post birth.

## 3. Chronic Stress and Anxiety

Any life left out of balance will eventually be reflected in the body. I recently saw a woman in her early twenties who told me that she had recently suffered burnout and was in a world of body pain not really knowing why. "For two years I kept telling myself, *It's okay. it's okay,* then I had a total meltdown at work over something really tiny."

Shocking but true. This level of sustained life pressure pulls and contorts our bodies out of balance so completely that everything begins to hurt. Her pelvis and her body reflected the imbalance in her life and had gradually become contorted and pain-filled. Stress makes us tense, and because we are stronger on our dominant side, the imbalance of the accumulating tension pulls and eventually locks us off-center. Subject to this chronic angulating pressure, the pelvis distorts, stopping where it gets stuck at the maximum twist of about 2.5 centimeters. Having reached its limit, the imbalance then radiates throughout the body, creating *painful proliferation*. If this physical decline happened suddenly, you would be shocked, but when it happens slowly, we learn to accept the incremental limitations.

The first sign is usually an aching lower back and a niggly hip on the same side, with a numb or painful area on the thigh. Next on the list is a hamstring that feels torn and sore. Sometimes a swollen knee and Achilles discomfort occurs, with plantar fasciitis developing last. On the way up comes lower back pain and a shoulder problem, possibly radiating into the arm usually on the opposite side to the hip pain. Then on upward to the neck and, lastly, headaches/migraines with possible dizziness and "fuzzy thinking." Our clothes, following any misalignment, provide useful reference points. If the zip on your jeans always heads off to one side, or your shirt buttons are not vertical, you're probably out of whack. The label on top of this model's foundations is crooked (see image overleaf). The four horizontal black lines show mild asymmetry through all four reference points, and the vertical line dissecting the label at the base of her spine almost touches the side of her left sneaker.

If stress is causing your "out of whackness," the painful areas in this image will switch on in order, beginning at the belt line. As exposure to stress continues, the discomfort spreads both up and down, away from the center. Responding to a reduction in stress, the pains will switch off in the reverse of this same sequence. Generally speaking, the younger and fitter you are, the faster you can recover, but age is no barrier. So far, my oldest client who made a complete recovery was ninety-three, and the youngest was three months.

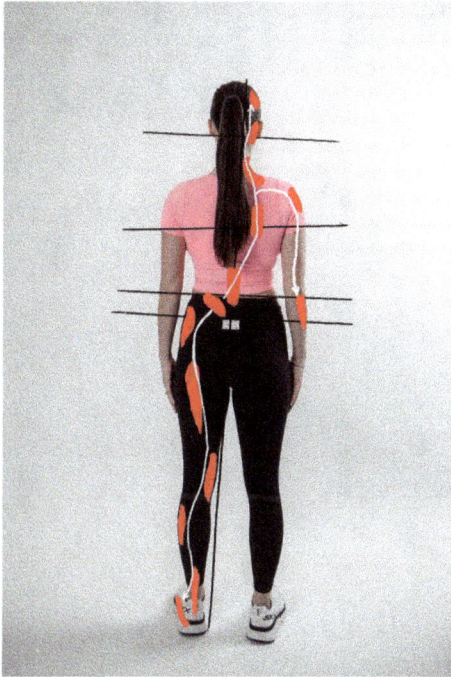

*The whack check introduced in this chapter needs to be adopted as an essential part of any routine health check.*

That pretty much covers why a twisted body gets so sore in so many different places. Now let's take a closer look at what can actually fail as a direct result of being out of whack.

# CHAPTER 2

# AVALANCHE OF FAILURES

## COMMON LANGUAGE

*"The rot is really starting to set in now."*
*"That's the way the cookie crumbles."*
*"It's all downhill from here."*

## QUICK FIX

A body left out of whack progressively deteriorates and can initiate any or all of the following: disc failure, bone deterioration, joint problems, mobility reduction, pain, nerve entrapment, blood vessel restrictions, muscle dysfunction, fatigue, and depression. Beginning with the whack check, restore functional alignment using "pulling your leg and sacral shifters" (Chapter 19, Repairs and Maintenance) daily.

A balanced relaxed body will suffer very little if any wear and tear as we age. Re-visiting the house analogy for a moment, you will know how easily doors and drawers move when their supporting structures are correctly aligned. This freedom to move puts no more force on individual components than each part's own weight. But have you ever been to a home where things were out of line? A misaligned door rapidly wears that tell tale arc, grooving through the carpet fibers or scraping the varnish off wooden flooring as it is dragged to open and close. Paint wears off the sides of drawers and hinges, giving in to the angulating pressures, wear at the shaft. Next to fail are the handles and catches. Over time, the exertion required to move these structures sees us either pulling out the screws or snapping off the handles.

Just like the house, short-term foundational misalignment in our bodies does not do a lot of damage. But leave anybody out of whack for an extended period of time and what we call the rot, really starts to set in. Standing, sitting, in fact any movement requires more effort than before. Even staying still with a bent body, requires our muscles to constantly hold on rather than just balance. This holding creates extra pressure, more than the individual components were designed to handle and just like the house, parts of our bodies wear out and break!

PETER (Like Mary, all my male clients will be referred to as Peter in this book.)

*Peter fell onto his left buttock ten years ago and had been in pain ever since. Following three years of medication, he was given experimental surgery to alleviate pressure from his sciatic nerve. The operation split the piriformis muscle located under the glutes, which can pressurize the sciatic nerve as it passes over, under, or sometimes even through. He said the surgery had helped—and so had his new $600 work chair—but the pain was now worsening and spreading from where it had always been in his lower back, down his leg, and into his foot. Furthermore, it was now traveling upward to include his opposite shoulder. Peter's initial assessment revealed the underlying reason for his ongoing discomfort and more recent deterioration. He had a pelvic rotation of 2.5 centimeters and was standing eight kilos more heavily on his left foot. Once the pelvis was returned to its correct alignment, and with the compensatory holding patterns released, Peter stood and walked a little hesitantly at first, pain-free.*

It's important to mention here that Peter's experience was not an instantaneous cure-all. Ten follow-up sessions were required to completely free his contorted body. The following list describes the path his body was heading down. Unresolved, he could have controlled his speed down this road to physical ruin, but the path itself does not change.

- Disc failure
- Bone deterioration
- Joint problems
- Mobility reduction
- Pain
- Wiring (nerves)
- Plumbing (blood vessels)
- Muscle dysfunction
- Fatigue
- Depression

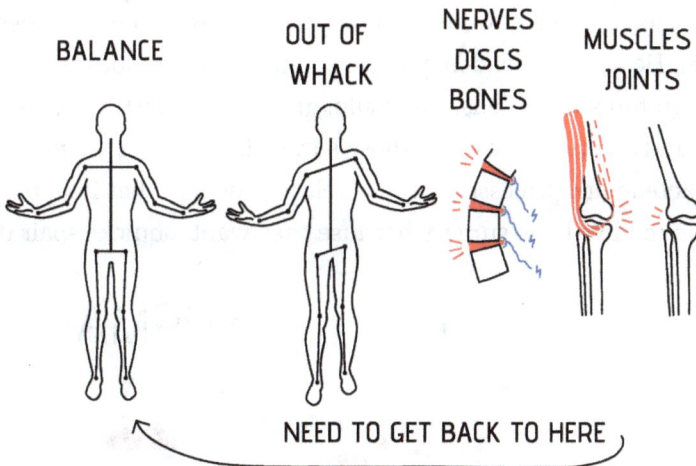

BALANCE    OUT OF WHACK    NERVES DISCS BONES    MUSCLES JOINTS

NEED TO GET BACK TO HERE

## DISC FAILURE

Discs are designed to evenly cushion the gaps between our spinal bones, allowing what would otherwise be a solid object to bend and slightly rotate. All of these movements need to be temporary because if we stay bent or rotated, we risk damaging the discs. Too much pressure on one side and an enlarged gap on the other creates squashing and tearing.

*Make a loose fist and rest the points of your knuckles firmly onto a hard surface like a table or bench. Applying the same pressure, angle your fist up on one side until only the knuckle of your index finger is making contact. You will instantly feel that the same pressure concentrated into this much smaller area hurts. This is the reality for any disc where the body weight is forced over onto one edge instead of being evenly distributed.*

Any muscle recruited to help support the imbalance does so by bracing. But this just makes everything tighter and generates more pain, making us more tense (pushing your knuckle harder onto the firm surface). It is this downward spiraling imbalance, pain, and tension that can destroy otherwise healthy components by collapsing discs, tearing the opening side, and forcing disc protrusions out on the compressed side.

Dr. Joe told me how he had chipped away at the current medical model. He said the tendency in that mindset was to look at patients through too small a lens. He would, given the opportunity, passionately and carefully challenge those surgical specialists he most often interacted with professionally. He relayed the fact that it suits some people to have back surgery because they want a quick repair done.

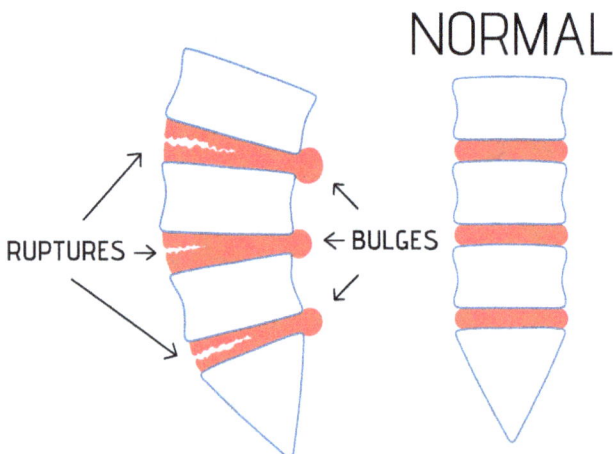

NORMAL

RUPTURES →    ← BULGES

But in the same breath he made it very clear that it was his firm view that surgery was mostly a *temporary* fix. He said that the twisting and tensioning pressures that brought about the individual component failure would, if left untreated, eventually cause breakdown at the next vertebral level. He then added that surgical interventions could have a far higher success rate once coupled with the realignment and balancing of the whole body. Dr. Joe also insisted that all patients scheduled for corrective spinal surgery should be X-rayed from the front while standing in front of a plumb bob as he felt this was the most reliable way to measure any structural anomalies.

## PETER

*Peter is the out-of-whack back model pictured in chapter one. He had three successful lower back surgeries over a ten-year period. But after two discectomies (removal of the part of the disc putting pressure on a nerve branch) and one L4-L5 disc fusion (surgically connecting the lowest two bones in the spine), Peter's back was in trouble again. Currently on three different drugs to manage nerve pain and inflammation, he was understandably distressed. The latest imaging revealed disc height reductions and disc protrusions pressurizing nerve branches at L2-L3 (the next two bones above the surgeries). During his initial session, as I began to adjust the alignment of his 2.5-centimeter out-of-whack pelvis, Peter had recall a serious motorcycle accident. "Thinking about it now, it was really quite violent, and my back has not been right since."*

## BONE DETERIORATION

If this uneven pressure is left for long enough (a decade or more), the bones of the spine will deteriorate. The side under the most pressure can begin to crumble, transforming the vertebrae into wedges rather than blocks. Some of this localized deterioration can be attributed to sustained mechanical pressure alone. The rest will be the result of

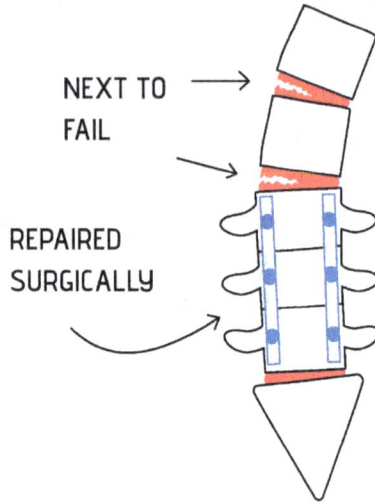

NEXT TO FAIL

REPAIRED SURGICALLY

pressure on tiny blood vessels stopping the blood from reaching those areas most compressed.

## JOINT FAILURE

Ever wondered why one hip or knee wears out first? If it was just normal wear and tear, they would both wear out at the same rate. Right? It's not that simple though. Our joints are easily capable of lasting a lifetime as long as they are lubricated, correctly aligned, and relaxed. With the pelvis higher on one side, the muscles around that one hip joint become tighter. This increased tension, once compacted, not

BONES CHANGE SHAPE

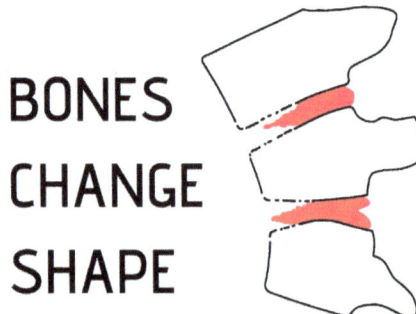

only restricts blood flow to the joint but forces the head of the femur too firmly into the socket, excluding lubrication, which dehydrates, crushes, and wears down the joint surfaces.

*To feel the difference that pressure and lack of lubrication can cause your hip, rub your finger and thumb together firmly. How many days do you think it will take before you rub through the skin? Once it's feeling raw, apply a single drop of cooking oil to the surface and continue to rub, only this time more gently. Get the idea? Ouch!*

## MOBILITY REDUCTION

Most people who have an out-of-whack lower back very quickly lose about half of their spinal function. Everything we could expect to do within the normal range pre-twist reduces by close to 50 percent. This makes it difficult to do things like reaching our feet or looking over our shoulders. The arms and legs start to shut down, too, but not evenly because there is more holding pressure on one side. But they do begin to weaken and stiffen. In the case of the legs, most people describe this feeling as having to "drag" their legs forward.

## PAIN

Wherever our bodies manage the imbalance, pain is generated to alert us to the problem. It begins as a low-level pain, then becomes agonizing if left untreated. The worst cases I have seen are when clients are scared to move and take several excruciating minutes just to get on or off the treatment table. In the words of my client "Mary," when asked to turn over, she replied, "Are you expecting that to be done today?"

## WIRING (Nerves)

Most of our nerves exit between the vertebrae. These exit points need to be big enough for the bones to move a little without putting any

# PRESSURE ON NERVES

pressure on the conductors. The muscles need to be *squishy* enough not to trap the nerve branches as they travel through, under, or over. This ensures their uninterrupted sending and receiving of the signals. If you have ever been in a cell phone dead zone, you will relate to how difficult it is to have a conversation without a clear signal. Likewise, our bodies require a constant 5G-like signal to and from the brain.

Once a nerve is compressed, it cannot operate correctly. An example of a healthy flow of information is: *switch on, switch off, ramp a little up, ramp a little down*. Under pressure, this can become: *s..tc. o., sw... h ..f, r..p a l...l..p, r..p . li...e d..n*. Imagine if your heart was receiving this gibberish. Even worse is the very real possibility of nothing but static: *shshshsshshshshshshshshshshshshsh*. This constant stimulation, devoid of clear instruction, is one of the major causes of muscle and organ failure.

## PLUMBING (blood vessels)

Every muscle that holds tension to manage the imbalance runs the risk of trapping blood vessels, reducing pressure and flow. This places any body component reliant on fully functional blood flow in a dire situation. I'm guessing you could easily relate to how difficult your life could be if your shower was dripping instead of fully flowing.

## MUSCLE DYSFUNCTION

Muscles called away from their normal day-to-day functioning to help manage the imbalance are recruited into the never-ending job of *holding*. Given the choice, no muscle would apply for this job. Sure, it is not complicated. All you have to do is stay switched on. But the single worst thing we can do to any muscle— bar cutting it or smacking it with a blunt object— is to leave it switched on as it will become progressively compacted, weakened, and very painful.

## FATIGUE

A lot of energy is wasted by trying to get a movement-restricted body to move. When getting out of bed, getting dressed, or getting into a vehicle becomes a major mission, it can wear down even the hardiest of souls. I have heard stories from many people who had to give up the activities they once enjoyed. One such man, although strong as an ox, was reduced to relying on his partner to put on his socks and shoes. Some have stopped running or quit sports altogether; others simply want to play with their grandchildren and be able to pick them up. Some clients (usually after they have recovered) described this feeling as one of pulling a concrete block behind them wherever they went. This persistent energy depletion can negatively impact our natural buoyancy, leading to *depression*.

## DEPRESSION

A decade ago, Peter, who had already received several remedial treatments and was well on his way to full recovery from his chronic back pain, bounded through my clinic door, proudly announcing that his children said, "Mister Grumpy is finally gone!" I think there is a strong link between chronic pain and depression. I don't mean that the cause of all depression is chronic pain, but if even the slightest movement amplifies your constant pain, it can feel like someone is following you around, poking you with a stick, wearing you down physically and mentally.

*Sit in a chair and have someone place their hands on your shoulders, holding you down and forward. In this position, try to feel relaxed, safe, positive, and happy. Then sit up freely as tall as you can and try to feel tense, insecure, negative and sad. It's as hard to feel down while upright as it is to be held forward and feel up. With no explanation for the discomfort and no solution in sight, and the overwhelming feeling that "this is as good as I am ever going to feel," it must be depressing.*

There may be some surprising revelations in this next chapter concerning a few of our popular ill-health misconceptions.

# CHAPTER 3

# DELVING A LITTLE DEEPER

## COMMON LANGUAGE

*"Looks like he's torn a hammstring."*
*"My bladder isn't what it used to be."*
*"Let's get to the bottom of it."*

## QUICK FIX

Living out of whack generates localized conditions currently viewed as isolated. This can result in causal misdiagnoses, raised or lowered arches, torn hamstring, leaky bladder, and calf strain to name just a few. Even concussion symptoms can be generated as a consequence of an out-of-whack foundation. Restore balance to the body, stretch, and gently exercise regularly to eradicate any out-of-whack initiated symptoms.

If you are suddenly woken in the night by a smoke alarm, do you remove the battery and go back to sleep, or do you heed its warning and get everyone out of the house? Of course, you say without hesitation, "Get out of the house! Don't grab any personal belongings. Alert the kids, grab the pets, get out quickly, and *stay out!*"

We all know that a smoke alarm is there to alert us to a developing situation that, if ignored, could maim us or even end our life. Thankfully, the importance of installing smoke alarms in our homes has been drilled into us, and we place them at strategic points. There is even an annoying beep that sounds to remind us to change the batteries when they are running low. Fires can very quickly spread through any home, blocking safe exit points within minutes of igniting. Thanks to these clever, inexpensive little gadgets, we can sleep in peace knowing full well that even if there is the slightest whiff of smoke, we will be instantly alerted. Likewise, if you get an alarm signal from your body, do you respond by investigating the source of something that could further harm you or, in the worst-case scenario, end your life? Or do you see the signal as a time-consuming inconvenience to be overridden and silenced any way you can?

We possess in each of our bodies a set of pain receptors and signaling equipment that would rival even the most saturated traffic monitoring and security network in the biggest cities around the world! So why would we think we know better and ignore a warning? Thanks to pharmaceuticals, we are able to keep "soldiering on" in spite of warning signals from our bodies. Modern medicine is wonderful, except when it assists us in harming ourselves. If we start to push ourselves a bit too hard and experience mild, medium, or even severe pain signals, we can choose a matching dosage of medication to silence our alarms and keep going. All I suggest is that you think about responding appropriately to emerging body pain instead of masking it.

Yes, I know it is terribly inconvenient for your body to start nagging that parts are failing because you are doing too much, especially when you "have so much more to do." I see a few clients whose inability to slow down even for a moment has them on my treatment table with the phone in hand, never disconnecting or taking the time to focus on the nature of true healing. You can intervene before a sore shoulder becomes frozen, an uncomfortable knee or hip needs replacing, or a tight back requires surgery. Start by taking full responsibility for what is actually happening in your life and, correspondingly, to your body. There are a couple of big switches inside us labeled *mind* and *body*. They only have two positions: on and off. It takes a lot of pressure for a long time to get either of them to move, but when they do it is calamitous. When any of these fires are left burning too long, they have the capacity to shut us down. If you choose not to stop, your body will eventually stop you.

# HAVE YOU REALLY TORN YOUR HAMSTRING?

Have you ever been watching football and seen one of the forwards grab the ball and suddenly sprint toward the try line only to leap onto one leg and hop to an agonizing halt, then hear from the commentator, "Ooh, that looks like a torn hammy"? There are, in fact, two possible scenarios here, both sharing the same initial cause. It could be a torn hamstring, but that player could also be feeling the leg referral from a rotated pelvic joint. I know, you may well be thinking, *Did you just say the hamstring may be okay, even though it's running red-hot and agonizingly painful?* The short answer is yes.

Suddenly rotating and locking the sacroiliac joint (SI joint) at the back of the pelvis refers a pain in the hamstring that feels just like a torn muscle. (Even the predictive text is struggling with this alternative to the common explanation by suggesting that I correct it to read: "refers to a pain in the hamstring.") With gradual onset, the discomfort developing in the leg is most often described as a sore muscle, but because of its instantaneous nature, this type of injury is more often than not diagnosed as a muscle tear.

## MARY

*Mary hobbled into my clinic, slightly bent forward, limping away from one very painful upper leg. "There is probably not much you can do for me. I've been told I have torn my hamstring." Mary's pelvis was out of whack to the max. After a thirty-minute session, and with her limp almost gone, she said, disbelievingly, that it felt "a lot better." She returned a week later having had her original diagnosis reaffirmed, in spite of an overall improvement of about 75 percent within seven days. Mary left at the end of that second thirty-minute session walking normally and pain-free.*

Mary had been feeling the agonizing referral from her rotated sacroiliac joint. Had it been a muscle tear causing the same level of pain, it would have taken several months to heal fully. Now, to turn this whole scenario on its head, if Mary had sprinted with her SI joint rotated, she could have actually torn her hamstring. As one side of the pelvis rotates and locks forward, it pulls both ends of the hamstrings farther apart. Our hamstrings travel about 3 centimeters from fully open to fully closed, most of which can be preloaded by a rotated pelvis. Fully extend these pre-tractioned muscles and they will tear!

## THE BACK AND HIP SWAP JOBS

If you are painfully out of whack, the muscles around one of your hips will respond by holding tight in a localized lockdown to protect it. As we run or walk, our legs (pre-injury) swing back behind us to about fifteen degrees past vertical. But this natural travel drops down to a staggering zero or, even worse, a hobbling less-than-zero reading as the muscles hold on to try and help. This stops your leg swinging, forcing your back to bend instead. This bending back and forth with every step can ruin an otherwise healthy back. You can see in the following images how the lower back is unaffected by the leg position in the image on the left and in the center. The shortened hip flexor becomes obvious in the right image as it pulls the lower back forward to allow the movement-restricted leg to travel past center. (This is explained more fully in Chapter 4.)

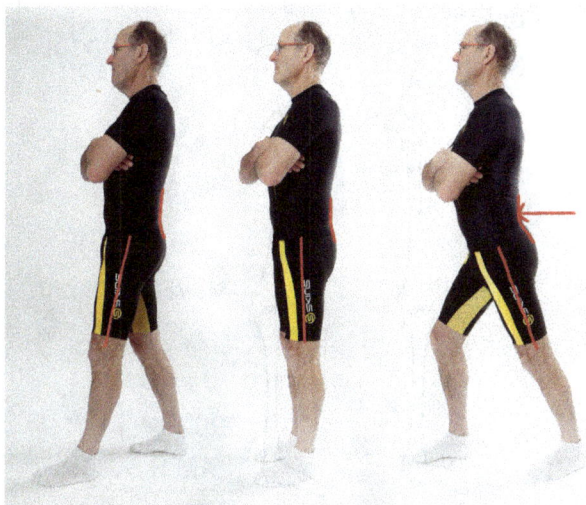

## HALF PENGUIN, HALF DUCK

Most ducks walk around with their bodies horizontal. This rotates both of their legs inwards. Emperor penguins stand vertically which rotates their legs outwards. The angle of our pelvis affects the position of everything below it in a similar way. Tilt it forward, like the horizontal-bodied duck, and the legs turn in. Rotate it backward and the

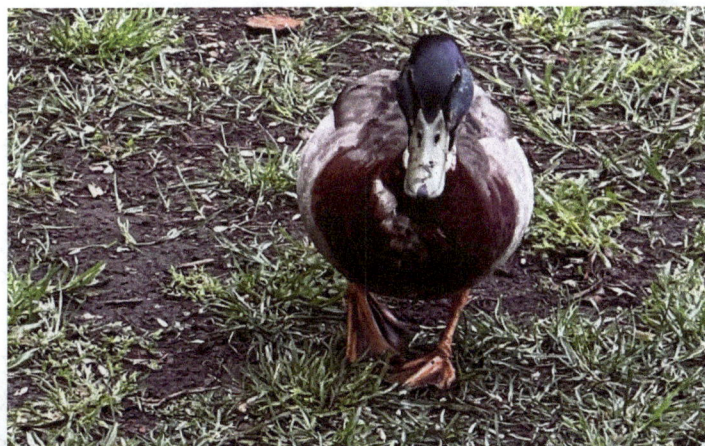

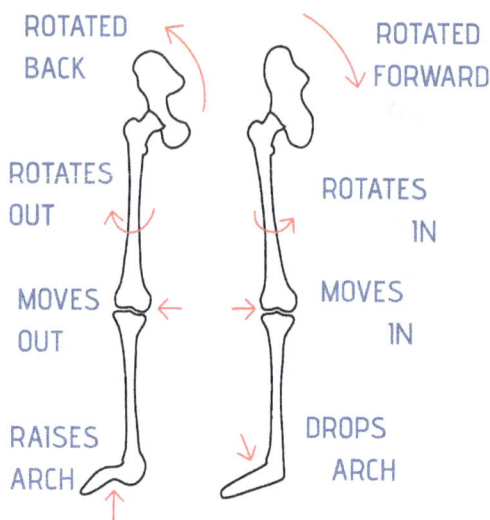

legs turn out with the front of our feet spread wide. Because any foundational rotation takes one side of our pelvis forward and the other back, we end up with one of each. This twists the ankle and knee joints in opposite directions, raising one arch while dropping the other.

## WEAK AT THE KNEES

With one leg turned in and the other out, both knee joint surfaces are misaligned. The weight transfers to the inner edge on one side and out on the other. The downward force focuses on a small point of each knee joint surface, eventually punching a hole in the cartilage or rupturing the meniscus. During the summer most people out walking are wearing shorts. This also means that knee braces are visible. There are a lot of them, and it is very rare to see one on a knee that is tracking in a straight line. If you are wearing a knee brace, get someone to video you walking from directly in front. You will more than likely see your knee move off-center as your body weight comes down onto your foot. In most cases, knee pain is signaling a knee that is tracking off-center below an out-of-whack pelvis.

## PETER

*Aged eighty-seven, he presented with lower back, right hip, and left neck pain. He showed me the heel raiser insert in his shoe to compensate for his recently (mis)diagnosed "short leg." Closer inspection revealed a pelvic rotation, giving Peter an apparent leg length difference of 2.5 centimeters. The heel raiser, while keeping his leg comfortably retracted on that side, had been keeping his pelvis twisted, making recovery impossible.*

## LIGHT-BULB MOMENTS

Switch a light on, and if the bulb is functioning properly, it lights up. Tennis elbow, golfer's elbow, and even carpal tunnel can all have their origins in our twisted foundations. It's the same as the previous scenario involving the neck, only this time the symptoms have radiated into a limb. I've chosen these three examples of what are commonly recognized as localized arm injuries, but anywhere along this path from our necks to the fingertips, or from our backs to our toes can be remotely affected. The constant out-of-whack pressure on blood vessels and nerves, although slight, reduces blood flow and radiates static into the unfortunate muscles of your arm (or leg). This only hurts in your elbow because that's where these tensioned muscles join to the bone. If you want the light to go out, then don't remove the bulb; instead, turn the switch off at the source. What I mean by that is if you have muscle pain anywhere in your body, check your spinal mobility first before treating the symptom. For example, golfer's elbow and tennis elbow are usually generated by the neck being a bit stuck at the base. If you have either of these, or even a frozen shoulder, a fairly safe bet is that your neck will not be able to turn your head to 90 degrees either way. Once you remedy your neck tension, restoring it to full mobility, your symptoms will have improved. Then, all that is left to do is a bit of localized limb treatment and stretching to restore full range to the muscle or muscles that were affected.

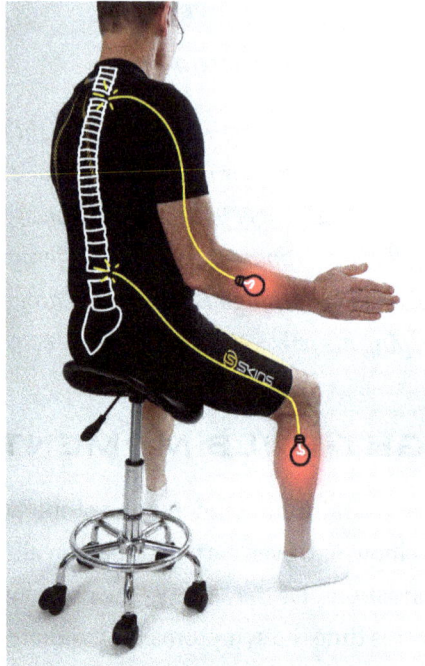

## MARY

*Unable to lift either of her arms past her shoulders and in constant pain, particularly when trying to sleep, Mary was diagnosed with bilateral rotator cuff injuries. This had been managed with yards of strapping tape covering her aching shoulders, and cortisone injections were offered as the most logical next step. The first thing I did was to remove all of the strapping. It looked very impressive and made her more comfortable in the short term, but it did not address the origin of her pain and dysfunction. Sure, Mary had lost most of the function in both of her shoulders, and the pain was often excruciating, but there was very little actually wrong with them. The problem was coming from her contorted upper-body light switches. She was totally out of whack, which was transferring the twisting and compaction into the base of her neck. After two restorative sessions with me, her stiffened ribs and neck gently remobilized, the light switches in her anterior neck muscles all turned off. Her shoulders*

*and arms responded to a little direct muscle and joint release, and*
*Mary's shoulders both returned to normal, pain-free function.*

## PETER

*"I need you to have a look at my bloody shoulder. It's pissing me off! I can't*
*sleep. You probably can't do much to help. I think it's buggered. I'm going*
*in for a cortisone jab in a couple of weeks," Peter complained. About fif-*
*teen minutes into the session, Peter's shoulder was pain-free and fully*
*mobile. All that was left was to show him how to continue self-treatment*
*at home by laying his shoulder pressure point on a cricket ball and mov-*
*ing his arm back and forth (see Chapter 19 for more detail). What had*
*been keeping Peter awake had been the agonizing light bulb on the front*
*of his shoulder. This had been referring from a muscle's pressure point on*
*his shoulder blade at the back, activated by a switch left on in his out-of-*
*whack neck. Another classic light-switch and light-bulb situation.*

## HORSES

How much of this can be applied to horses? The short answer is, all of
it. A telltale sign of active referrals in humans is a troublesome big
toenail or two. Horses walk on four hooves that originally began as
toenails.

If your horse is lame, look away from the hoof for the cause.

## TEETH AND GUMS

Your teeth and gums are at the mercy of your neck in a similar way.
There are two pressure points, one either side of your spine, beside
your shoulder blades. If the base of your neck goes "out" or gets too
tight, these pressure points will fire up, sending inflammatory referrals directly into your jaws. If you are having trouble with inflamed
gums, tooth sensitivity or have even lost a tooth, the original problem

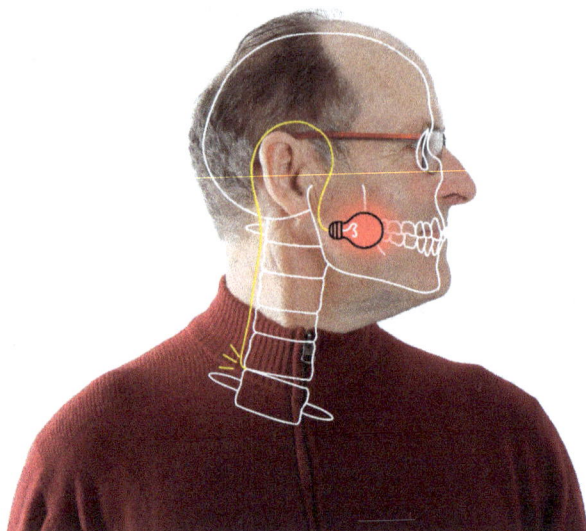

may still be there, a long way from your symptoms and under most peoples' radar. Make sure your neck is fully mobile pain-free and have the pressure point activity resolved to eliminate any referrals. Then your teeth and gums can resume normal operation, undisturbed.

## CONCUSSION

Concussions are surprisingly common. Sixty-nine million sports-related concussions occur worldwide annually. Clearly, some concussions are the direct result of impact on the brain, but others are not. The human brain is protectively cushioned, floating in a bath of cerebrospinal fluid. This liquid maintains a little space between the very soft, easily damaged brain and the rigid, bony, impact-resistant skull. This liquid's ability to flow protects the brain by absorbing the shock of low impact bumps to the head. But hitting the head at speed against a solid object displaces this liquid, bringing the front of the brain into contact with the inside surface of the skull. Without this insulating protective layer of fluid, the brain receives the full collision impact. Because of this, it makes perfect sense to look at concussion purely as a brain impact injury. But there is another possible scenario. One that is potentially much more significant in terms of the back half of the brain's ability to function normally long term. As long as the head and body are traveling forward at the same rate the neck is relatively safe. But if you stop the head with the rest of the body still traveling forward, the neck becomes an injury site. These neck injuries can reduce blood flow to significant sections of the brain. I know based on my years of building hot rods, the futility of mismatching engine and fuel supply. Replacing a four-cylinder, forty-eight horsepower engine with a four hundred eighty horsepower V8 had to include a total upgrade of the fuel supply system to match the new engine. Had I expected the new, bigger engine to run on the original fuel supply, one-tenth of its requirements, it would have coughed and spluttered, performing very poorly, if at all. This scenario relates directly to concussion-related neck injuries where the brain can be forced into operating with greatly reduced blood supply.

## PETER

*Having assisted Peter's return to running, he was hopeful I could make a difference for his son, who had been diagnosed with an incurable concussion two years prior. Peter Junior's symptoms looked strikingly similar to those I had been successfully treating for years: headaches, nausea, dizziness, sleeplessness, fatigue, poor balance, mild depression, and photophobia. Close inspection revealed him to be 2.5 centimeters out of whack with severely compacted soft tissue and joint misalignment throughout his entire upper rib cage and neck. A comparatively short block of sessions resolved his out-of-whack body and restored neck function, clearing out not just some but all of Peter Junior's symptoms!*

There are two large arteries rising off the heart that go directly to the front of the brain. The one you can see in the next image is much smaller in comparison and is the left of two equals in our necks. They are threaded up through holes in the vertebrae, which exposes

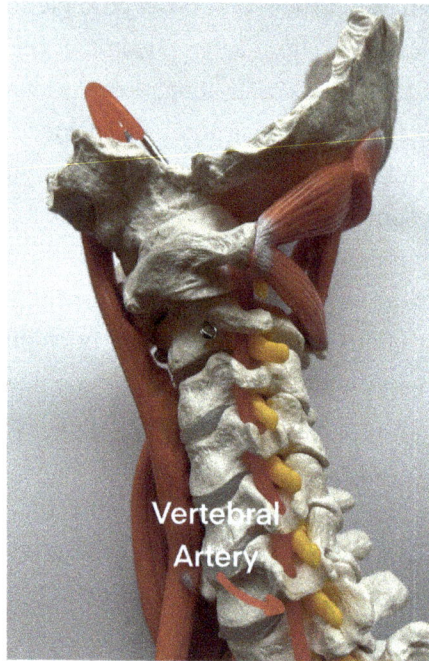

them to blockages from misaligned neck bones or direct pressure from the impact-damaged muscles. Together they supply the entire rear of the brain, the cerebellum, and the brainstem. Listed are their major functions:

| | |
|---|---|
| **Brainstem:** | breathing, consciousness, blood pressure, heart rate, sleep |
| **Cerebellum:** | muscle control, balance, movement |
| **Brain posterior:** | planned movement, spatial reasoning, attention, vision, auditory, sensory |

In the first image, everything is normal. The second image depicts localized muscular compaction, sandwiching the vertebral artery against the vertebrae, restricting or possibly even blocking blood flow.

The shrinking of the rear of the brain is, of course, unproven, but impaired blood flow must (at the very least) reduce its ability to function.

*You will already be aware of how this reduction in pressure and flow can affect whatever is on the receiving end. Picture one of your children standing on the hose that connects to your lawn sprinkler. Imagine it stopping and starting again once they take their foot off.*

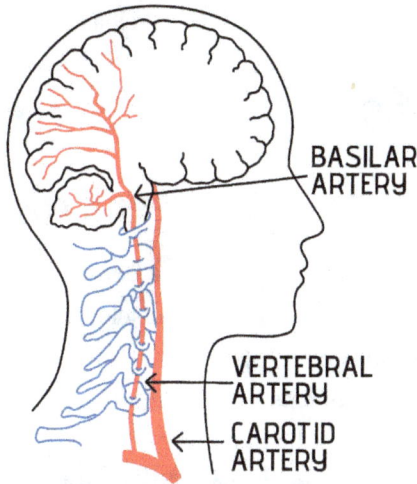

BASILAR
ARTERY

VERTEBRAL
ARTERY

CAROTID
ARTERY

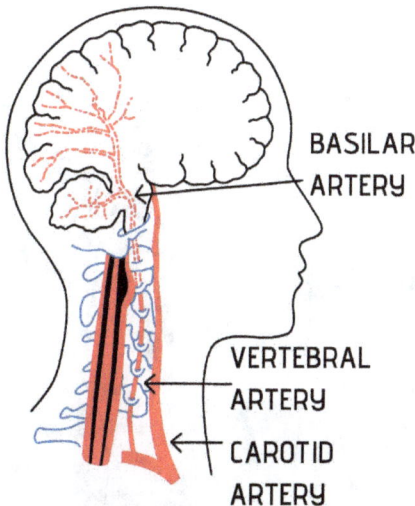

BASILAR
ARTERY

VERTEBRAL
ARTERY

CAROTID
ARTERY

A series of knocks to the head can be enough to cause the verte-brae to misalign and the neck muscles to compact, potentially block-ing both vertebral arteries. If you are inadvertently carrying this injury, you could pass out by simply turning your head to look over your shoulder or tipping your head backward to look up. (In the case of totally blocked vertebral arteries, some blood would still flow through from the carotid via the communicating arteries inside the head, but these are tiny in comparison.) To restore blood flow, simply resolve any out of whackness first, then release the neck. If you have a concussion diagnosis from your doctor, do the neck range of motion checks listed in Chapter 15.

## LIGHT BLADDER LEAKAGE

As the out-of-whack twisting pressure comes onto the L5-S1 nerve branch (base of the lower back), the muscle holding the urine in the urethral tube can lose clear operational signals.

Correct operation of this tiny doughnut-shaped muscle is essen-tial for keeping us dry. As the reduced nerve function makes it weaker, some of the urine is allowed to pass. This does not mean anything is

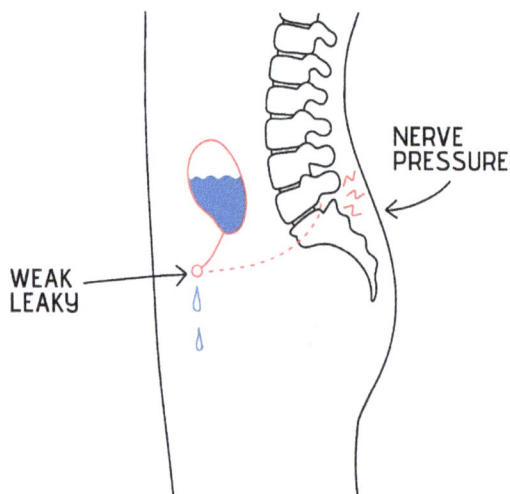

wrong with the bladder; it just has a weakened, leaky tap. Another unpleasant side effect may be a reduction in flow. Two female clients just this past week have reported a return to normal urine function after only a couple of sessions to alleviate their out-of-whack pelvis.

## WOULD YOU PUT AIR INTO A FLAT TIRE?

A slowly deflating tire can be a pain. Since it's not totally blown out, you don't need to replace it straight away, right? You could keep it going if you put more air in, but you'd you have to do this *every time* you go out! It's not something you would keep doing for long because it would be nonsensical. Likewise, by treating any of your out-of-whack body symptoms without rectifying the original cause, you are doing just that to your body.

Let's say it's your neck that's the problem. Your posture is pretty good, and your work station has been set up by the occupational therapist, but it keeps getting really sore on that one side! You go to the walk-in massage at the mall for a neck rub every second Wednesday, which feels great for a while, only to have the pain and stiffness return by Friday afternoon. The truth is, even if you had a neck rub every day, the problem would not stay away. The only way to stop your tire going down is by having it repaired. Eliminate the actual cause by remedying your out-of-whack body. There are several self-treatments listed in Chapter 19 designed specifically to get you back from being out of whack.

Departing from structural causes of dysfunction now, let's move forward and address that scary elephant in so many back-pain-filled rooms: emotions.

CHAPTER 4

# BACK PAIN USUALLY STARTS IN THE FRONT

## COMMON LANGUAGE

*"It was gut wrenching!"*
*"I felt it in the pit of my stomach."*
*"I took it all on board."*

## QUICK FIX

*Our psoas muscles, invisible to us, became mechanically preloaded and forced to work around a corner as our species evolved from crouching to standing. Further tractioning through emotional holding strangles the lower vertebrae from the inside, radiating discomfort and deterioration into the lower back. If you have back pain, stretch the muscles in your front, the hip flexors.*

Take a big breath and see how long you can hold it. You probably had to let it go somewhere between thirty seconds and two minutes. Keep repeating this for one thousand years and you may be able to match the deep-sea freediving Bajau people of Southeast Asia. Their spleens now carry enough extra oxygenated blood to allow the super-human feat of diving for thirteen minutes to a maximum depth of

STANDING            CROUCHING

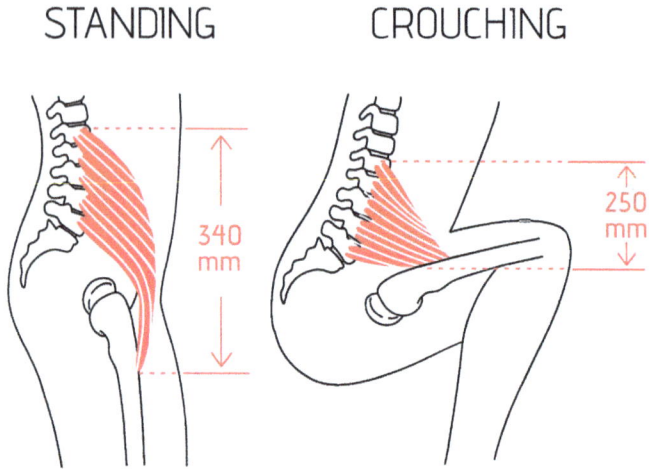

sixty meters (nearly two hundred feet). Our bodies have also adapted over time, allowing us to stand vertically.

In the very early stages of our evolution, humans spent most of their time with their hips flexed. A high percentage of our DNA (98.5 percent) is identical to chimpanzees,[1] and they still sit and crouch the way we used to. They don't stand up very often, but when they do, their short hip flexors keep their legs slightly bent. Thanks to our ancestors' efforts, we have now evolved to the point where we can stand up straight for prolonged periods.

Eons ago as we all transitioned from crouching to standing, this group of large muscles that used to operate horizontally in their mid-range were forced to follow the leg bone down around a corner into their new end of range at a near-vertical position. Our glutes have done the mirror image of this, transitioning into a movement that forces the muscles to bunch up behind us as they run out of a room. This pre-stretching of the hip flexors sets us up for most of our back problems. Shortening this muscle group by a centimeter or two while crouching does nothing noticeable because there is plenty of slack. Doing the same shortening while standing, pulls and holds the lower back forward because in this new position there is no slack. This introduces static tension and pressure. But what could cause these muscles to shorten again after all of that lengthening over centuries? The answer? Emotions.

## EMOTIONS

Most new clients present for their first appointment at my clinic with a back injury story explaining the physical trauma that caused their injury. As treatment progresses, another possible scenario always emerges. This is usually a recall of emotionally significant events. I never prompt anyone to tell their story of traumatic memories; these usually surface as the holding is released.

### EXAMPLE ONE
- "I did a bit of gardening last week. My back started to get really sore, and now I can't seem to stand up straight."
- Then, partway through the session I'll hear them add to the story: "We had our old family dog put down last week after a long illness."

### EXAMPLE TWO
- They'll swear: "All I did was step in a tiny wee dip in the lawn, and my back was in instant agony."
- About two treatments later, the client will add details of their personal life: "I'm going through a bit of a tricky time at the moment. I found out that my partner is cheating on me."

Physical strain being the primary contributing factor in back injuries is currently universally accepted throughout the commercial model. It's not really all that surprising though, under our present system in New Zealand of accident claims needing a physical (not emotional) cause. *Maybe it's time to include emotionally significant events into physical injury claims . . .*

## THE STRAW THAT BROKE
## THE CAMEL'S BACK

The lumbar spine is superbly engineered, incredibly tough, and well-constructed. The lower five vertebrae collectively weigh as much as the rest of the spine combined. I recently treated a retired farmer for a shoulder problem, and we got chatting about lifting heavy objects. He said they used to think nothing of lugging sacks of grain up to shoulder height to empty them into the seed drill hoppers. These sacks weighed approximately eighty kilograms each (about 175 pounds), and every year he would load enough of them to plant the whole farm. This was happening right across the country. So why is it that a person bending slowly forward to pick up a bar of soap weighing about 100 grams can severely injure themselves when their backs are made of the same stuff? The answer again? Emotions.

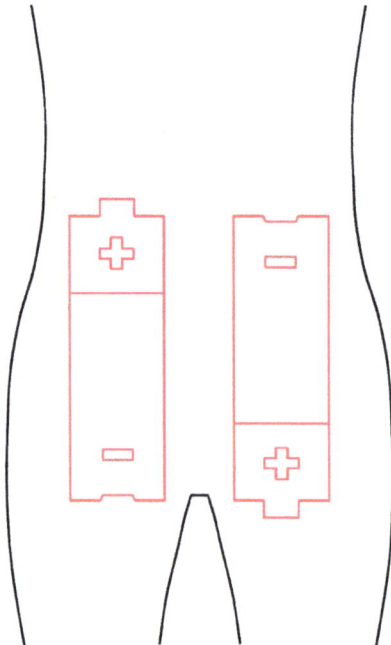

## GUT FEELINGS

*These mindful iliopsoas muscles form our emotional batteries* (see diagram on previous page). Because overload has become a reasonably acceptable part of our society, we have learned to containerize our feelings. It is both stress and our reactive anxiety that generate emotion, so I have decided to link them together throughout as *stress* and *anxiety*. This soft-tissue emotional reservoir allows us to put our current feelings on hold and carry on. If you have a fear of heights and have stood too close to the edge of a big drop, you may have felt your own "gut response." Having this storage facility available allows us to "suck it up."

## "OH, JUST SUCK IT UP!"

According to the Law of Conservation and Mass, matter can change form but is neither created nor destroyed. Therefore, unresolved feelings require either active processing or controlled storage. Emotion (energy in motion) potentially has enough power to make us uncontrollably violent or remarkably strong. In one recorded case, it was possible for a man to lift a car off an accident victim.[2] Presented with any stressful situation where the emotional surge is more than we can handle in the moment, we tend to pack it all away. We can even "swallow down feelings" that are too extreme to deal with. This includes all of the stuff we never express at work, at home, or socially—pretty much any situation in which you have been triggered and remained silent. Anything from "That guy is such an asshole. I'm sure one day somebody will tell him!" to "I just can't deal with this right now because I am too busy being busy," right through to being the recipient of the worst kinds of physical and or emotional abuse. These interactions all generate a reaction of excess energy that needs to be expressed or stored. By witnessing any situation where we can't or won't react in the moment, we inadvertently pack the feelings into our core muscles, our hip flexors. Our response in not expressing a feeling becomes a problem for us when we need to keep it where it is.

## KEEPING IT THERE

Any emotional energy that is not effectively held will escape and head back out into the world. This leakage has the potential to appear anytime, anywhere, so we need to constantly *keep a lid on it*. The last thing any of us needs in the middle of our chaotic lives is to have an untimely public meltdown. Unfortunately, the only effective form of emotional containment readily available is via muscular tension. Not the transitional type though. This muscle holding has to be strong and constant. Ever wondered why so many of us have a weak core? The holding required to manage stored emotional energy can involve such a large portion of these muscles that there are very few fibers left to do physical work.

*Grab a single piece of cutlery from the drawer, lightly toss it around a bit, then place it on the counter. Next, with the same hand closed and held tightly into a fist, try to pick it up again. Impossible! Totally distracted by the clenching, and literally unable to lift a finger, your hand has lost its ability to perform even this most basic of tasks.*

Your clenched fist is a pretty accurate representation of an emotionally charged core. Because it is extremely difficult to hold tension while moving, we completely withdraw our breathing from the abdominal area, forcing it up toward our neck (see Chapter 10). The entire breathing therapy industry focuses on returning our breath to a lower-body emotional storage facility. Because this reservoir is located out of sight and is energetically behind closed doors, we are allowed to pretend that it is not there. Imagine if it were to be stored in another more visible area of our bodies. Say, for example, on the top of our head. If this were the case, we would expect it to be noticed and even monitored by others. Then our *emotional baggage*, being on public display, would undoubtedly invite unsolicited feedback, such as,

"That must have been a difficult run-in with your boss." Or, "What's going on, you've got a new bulge up top." Or, "Oh dear, you must be having trouble at home again." Thankfully, this is not the case and we can keep functioning reasonably well on the outside while pretending that everything is tickety-boo on the inside.

## NOW THE DOWNSIDE

*Sit on one of your hands on a fairly firm surface. By keeping your hand squashed, it will go through stages of discomfort on its way to shutting down. After a minute or two, take your hand out and watch as it fires up again.*

How do you think your hand might look after one week, one month, or even a year? Shockingly, it's not unusual for this amount of bone-strangling, disc-compressing lower body tension to have been held in these muscles attached to the front of the lower back for a decade or two.

*Do a quick check of the charge held in your own batteries by standing upright with your side view visible in a mirror. Being careful not to tilt your back while moving only your leg closest to the mirror, see how far it swings back. Anything less than fifteen degrees past vertical indicates you are holding tension in your emotional storage muscles.*

*You can feel any stored tension by laying your hands on your hips and pressing your thumbs toward the inside of your pelvic bones. If it feels soft, then you're probably not holding on too much, but they can feel like a brick wall, in which case you are truly "full of it."*

As already mentioned in Chapter 3, anything less than the expected fifteen-degree leg extension or palpable pressure in the hip flexors will be strangling your lower back. Possible side effects of this pressure include:

- Lower back pain
- Gluteal collapse
- Reduction in lumbar flexibility

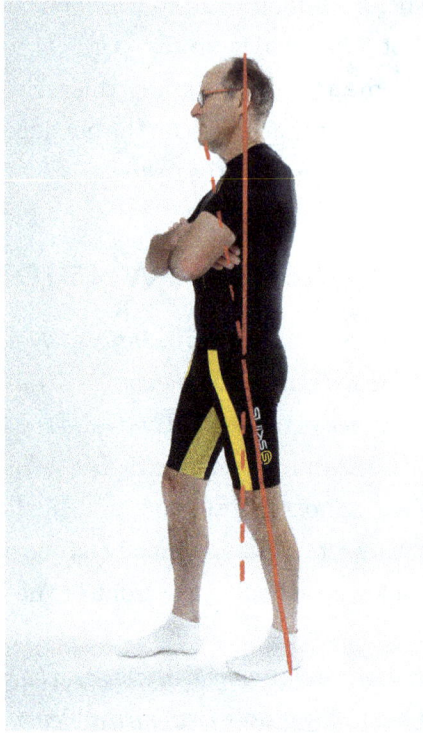

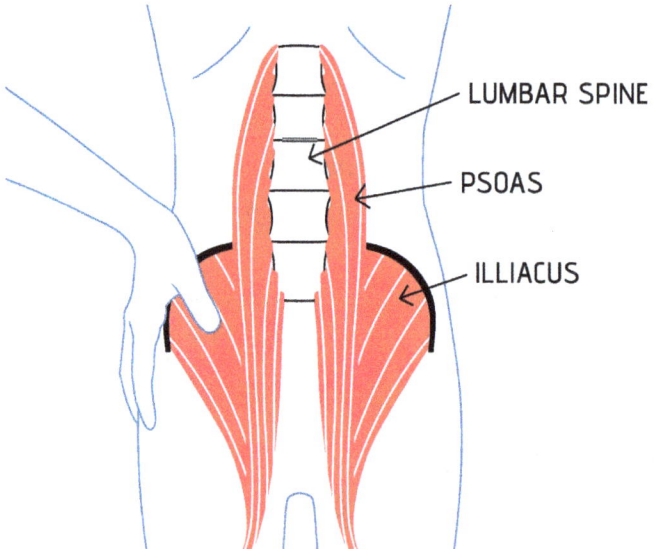

LUMBAR SPINE

PSOAS

ILLIACUS

- Strangulation of lumbar vertebrae
- Reduction in hip flexor strength
- Reduction in hip flexor length
- The back becomes like a hip joint
- Compression of disc cartilage
- Organ compression within the abdominal cavity
- Inflammation
- Constriction of major blood vessels
- Restricted lymphatic fluid flow
- Varicose veins in the legs
- Compromised lumbar nerve function

- LOWER BACK PAIN

A tow rope attached to and pulling a heavy object will wear at the points of contact. In a similar way, any muscle holding static tension will cause deterioration and generate pain where it is joined to the skeleton. In the case of the hip flexor group, this just happens to be across the belt line and in the center of the lower back up to the bottom of the rib cage. Although the original problem is in the front, we call it *back pain* because that is where these attachments are and that is where we feel it.

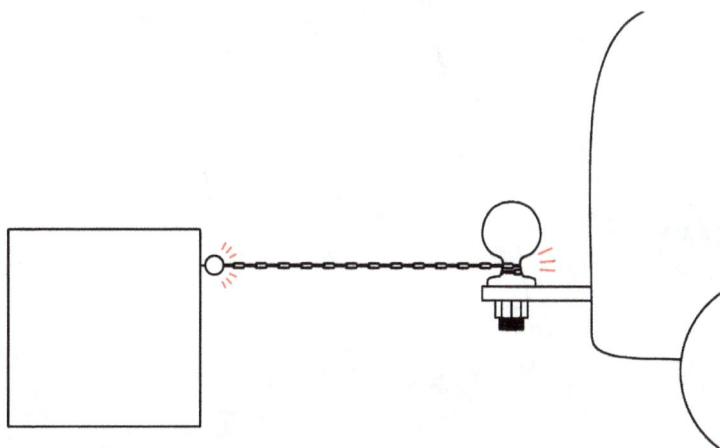

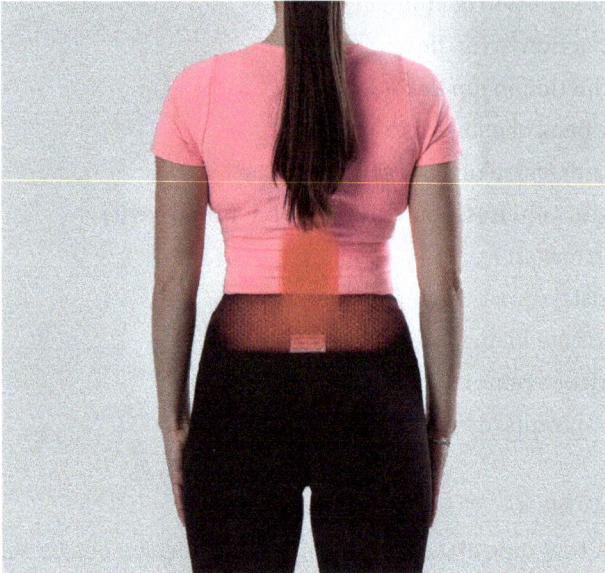

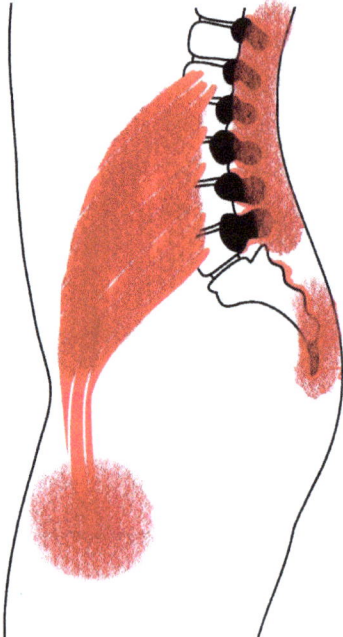

The other potentially painful attachments are on the inside top of the leg, which places a strain on your tailbone. You could be woken by either of these, or by a leg cramp on the inside of your thigh, if you have been worrying in your sleep.

- GLUTEAL COLLAPSE

As long as we are gathering and holding tension in our hip flexors, we are unwittingly taking the power away from our glutes. I have lost count of the number of clients who have said, and I quote, "I've been told I need to strengthen my glutes." I wonder how anyone could strengthen a muscle group that is switched off? Trust me when I say I have seen plenty of glutes (hip extensors) re-energized without the need for any specific exercises once the iliopsoas (comprised of two muscles: the iliacus and psoas major, which we call the hip flexors) is released. Reciprocal inhibition controls the level of stimulus available to muscle groups opposing each other. As one ramps up, the opposing one is forced to ramp down. So if you want to stop being what we call "half assed" and get your glutes back again, release your hip flexors!

- REDUCTION IN LUMBAR FLEXIBILITY

A relaxed lumbar spine will quite happily flex and extend every day throughout our whole life without damage. Once strangled, it becomes rigid, exposing it to injury. *Bend a glue stick and a pencil in both hands at the same time. You will get it the instant the pencil snaps.*

It probably requires quite a leap of faith to believe that a group of muscles can hold onto enough emotional energy to make them as hard as this pencil, (see overleaf). But they can and do. Once contracted and held, they can completely immobilize an otherwise supple lower spine.

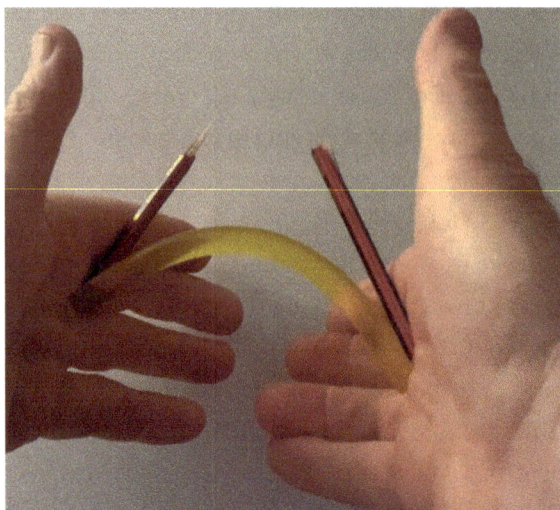

- REDUCTION IN HIP FLEXOR STRENGTH

  PETER: *"Tough guys walk with their shoulders."*

  You know the walk? It's the one done with hands in pockets, swinging the shoulders alternately to drag the legs forward. We just did the exercise where you can't even pick up a piece of cutlery with a clenched fist. These guys, commonly called *dropkicks*, have to swing their bodies to drag their legs forward as they walk to compensate for hip flexor weakness. (I'm guessing the name must have come from dropkicking being seen as a weakness when compared to going for a try.)

- REDUCTION IN HIP FLEXOR LENGTH

  Contracting your open hand into a fist shortens it, and so it is for your hip flexors. The shortening of these muscles is in direct proportion to the amount of emotional energy stored. This latent compression makes standing up and walking progressively more difficult.

- WHEN THE BACK BECOMES A HIP JOINT

  The lower back is forced into moving more to compensate for loss of movement at the hip joint (see Chapter 1, Out of Whack).

- STRANGULATION OF LUMBAR VERTEBRAE

    Because these powerful hip flexors are mounted on either side of the lumbar spine, they apply steadily increasing pressure against either side of the bones, reducing localized blood flow. Although very little blood flow is required to maintain any bone, if allowed to continue, this constant localized pressure will eventually result in deterioration of the vertebrae.

- COMPRESSION OF DISCS

    If you have ever seen the close-up, slow-motion action of a squash ball hitting a wall, you will know that they go almost flat upon impact! In spite of this, they last a surprisingly long time. But try putting one under the leg of a sofa for a while and it will rapidly rupture. Spinal discs perform in much the same way. As long as the pressures are transitional, they remain undamaged. The compression exerted by tensioned hip flexors is comparable to squeezing the discs in an engineer's vice and walking away. Of course, this would cause them to collapse and rupture.

- ORGAN COMPRESSION WITHIN THE ABDOMINAL CAVITY

    These four muscles (two psoas and two iliacus), once fully activated, can take up to half of the available space in the lower abdominal cavity!

    I am holding back on detail here, but I think it's fair to say that anything squeezed into this reduced space could easily become blocked, pushed out of shape, glued together, or strangled to such a degree that it could fail to function at all.

- INFLAMMATION

    A safe assumption here is that these muscles and the surrounding tissues would all become inflamed, as is generally the case with any muscle locked into contraction. Have you ever had the misfortune of being stuck in a space where the heat is blasting and you

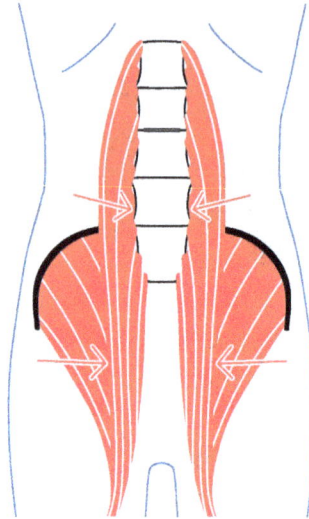

can't escape? The sort of situation I am talking about here is one like being in the passenger's seat of a car on a long journey when the driver insists on a hotter air con temperature than you. Your artificially overheated, sweatiness would rapidly change your body chemistry as the stress of the environmental change and lack of control kicked in. With these four muscles constantly running red hot, everything else that shares the abdominal cavity, blasted with inflammatory heat would also inflame. On the lower end of the scale is Cheer Leaders' Hip, where raising your leg diagonally across your body produces pain at the crease in your pants in front of the hip joint. Emotionally inflamed hip flexors produce pain at this location as the tendon passes through the groin. At the top end of the scale is Endometriosis (a disease of the uterus where the cause is currently listed as unknown).

- CONSTRICTION OF MAJOR BLOOD VESSELS

Blood flow to our lower extremities travels up and down in between the psoas major muscles. A pressure bulge (aortic aneurysm) can form in the artery wall directly above where it would get

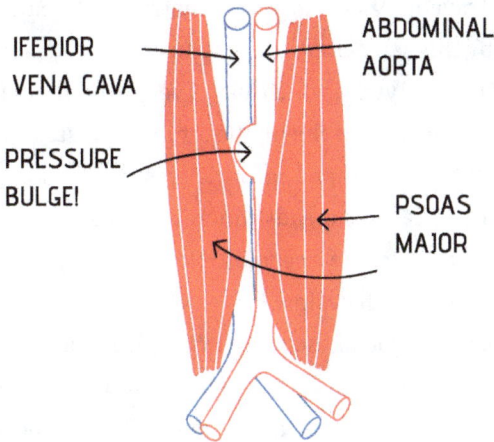

squashed were these two muscles left "switched on." The causes are listed as high blood pressure, smoking, atherosclerosis, and high cholesterol. What's missing here is direct mechanical pressure.

- RESTRICTED LYMPHATIC FLUID FLOW

Lymphatic fluid returning from the legs to the central body does not have a closed tubing pressure assisted return system like our veins do. Rather, it depends on pressure changes from within the body mostly generated by functional breathing. A series of open drains in the lymphatic return tubing located at strategic points around the body collect the fluid for reuse. These drains operate in a similar way to the drain in a household bath. You will know already that if the plug is left in, the water will not flow down the drain. These muscles share the groin space with our lower body drains for this semi-clear liquid. Of course the extra pressure and the lack of space the pressure causes will negatively affect their ability to operate

- VARICOSE VEINS IN THE LEGS

Varicosing of leg veins is widely accepted to be caused by failure of the veins themselves, but what if it's not their fault? These venous returns traveling back into the central body can become compressed by this same muscular expansion. The groin, a pinch point, is pretty tight anyway, which leaves very little room for movement. Once static tension in the hip flexor group restrict venous return, blood still being pumped into the legs can no longer pass easily back up the line. This steadily increasing volume will expand and possibly even rupture the multiple, single-direction fluid gates contained within the veins.

Another example of the same principle is the vein that becomes varicosed on the inside of the lower leg. You can see in the diagram how both vein and artery pass through a hole in the adductor muscle. This is the point where static muscular tension can pinch the vein, reducing blood flow back from the lower leg. I had one of these developing on my leg and—remembering my mother's painful experience rehabilitating from leg vein removal—decided to stretch it out before it deteriorated to the state of the one pictured overleaf. It worked. Doing the "you're so vein" leg stretch (see Chapter 19)

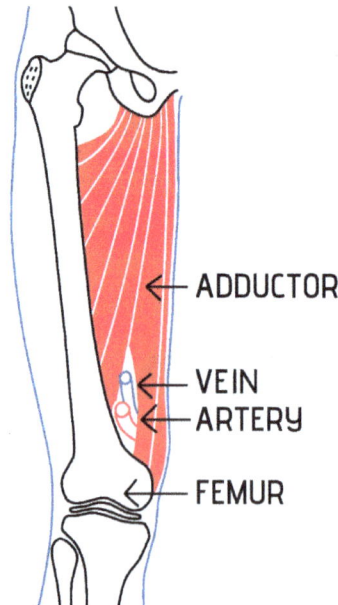

ADDUCTOR

VEIN
ARTERY

FEMUR

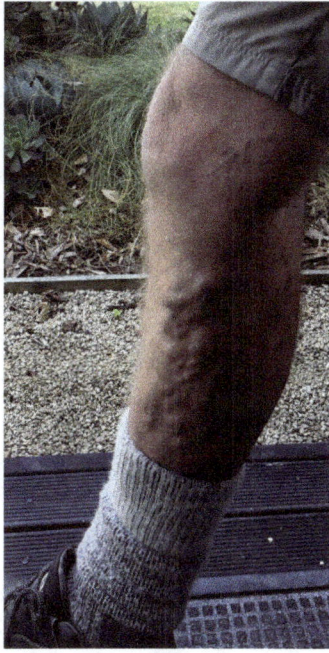

could save your life. Deep vein thrombosis (DVT), usually fatal, is caused by a blood clot dislodging, usually from the lower leg, that travels up to the lungs where it blocks the blood supply. These bulges in the lower leg veins are where some of those blood clots can form.

In this example, the lower leg is nowhere near the hip flexors, but the same principles can be transferred up to the abdominal region. Any pressure on blood vessels either coming or going has the potential to cause expansion in the walls of veins and rupturing of the non-return gates.

- COMPROMISED LUMBAR NERVE FUNCTION

Sciatica is the most widely recognized issue with compressed lumbar nerve function, but any nerve subject to this kind of sustained mechanical pressure will malfunction and let you know about it! The term *sciatica* is often misused. It is not unusual for clients to tell me that they have a long history of sciatica while holding their hand on the hamstrings of their right leg. These upper leg pains are usually only muscular. True sciatica involves an agonizing nerve entrapment affecting the entire sciatic nerve that runs from the pelvis all the way down the back and side of the leg, wrapping under the base of the heel.

## PETER

*A serious young man with a history of lower back problems, and more recently sciatica, presented with severely shortened psoas muscles and a pelvis that was 2.5 centimeters out of whack. He reported that for as long as he could remember, he'd always had back pain; it was only the intensity that varied. Returning to his fifth session, he announced with his first, albeit slightly wry smile that what I had already done for him was magic! When questioned about his use of the word magic, he replied that yes, most of his pain was gone and he was finding moving around so much easier. But somehow I had been able to lower the angle of the rear-view mirror in his car and totally rearrange the settings on his work chair without leaving my clinic.*

Time to transition to a subject we are all very familiar with but collectively choose to ignore or deny: being in a state of unrest. The unpleasant fact is that an uneasy mind rapidly spreads unease throughout our bodies, manifesting in system breakdowns.

# CHAPTER 5

# DISEASE: A STATE OF UNREST

## COMMON LANGUAGE

*"I'm walking on eggshells."*
*"She's stewing in her own juices."*
*"I'm not anxious, I just worry a lot."*

## QUICK FIX

If you have an outward leadership style that is weak and fragile, tyrannical and oppressive, or considerate and consultative, then that is also going to be reflected inward and will affect your general well-being, or lack thereof. If you are feeling disturbed or uneasy, take a moment to consider whether or not you have been listening to the signals your body is sending you. If your personal body leadership lacks integrity, your ill health is likely to continue or worsen. Don't be too rigid with personal improvements though. If you sometimes fall off the wagon with things like not doing your exercises every day or you eat a bit of junk food occasionally, it just means that you are normal.

Take a moment to think about your community. Do those controlling the space in which you live instill security or anxiety? When your significant other enters a room, are you more relaxed or on edge?

When you were a child, did your parents sustain a reassuring environment with firm, fair, trustworthy boundaries, or did they create one where you felt uneasy? Was the community in which you grew up safe, or were you constantly on edge? Throughout history, kings and queens have had the responsibility of law and order. As long as the king or queen's head was still firmly fixed to their shoulders, everyone in subservience could relax in the knowledge that if there was any trouble, it would be dealt with by them directly (or their representatives), and everyone in the kingdom would be kept reasonably safe. Chaos very rapidly sweeps through any community when the leader is absent, ineffective, or dies. Unfortunately, we have many homes, communities, and countries where the one who is the leader and is supposed to be instilling a feeling of safety and security for all of the occupants does anything but that. Aotearoa, New Zealand, has the highest domestic violence rates in the OECD (out of thirty-eight developed countries). Apparently, when the all Blacks suffer a significant loss, the Women's Refuge Center fills up overnight. Their 2023/4 report[1] states that 399,447 bed nights were delivered in that year.

## THE LION ON THE ROCK

The male lion never seems to do much. While the females do all of the hunting, he just lies there in the shade. He is, however, the head of security. Having earned his place, his life is on the line should anything go wrong. This means that the whole pride can relax as long as he is there. This same strength emanates from quietly confident people who mostly go unnoticed, but something about the *true strength* of their manner relaxes everyone around them.

## THE WIZARD OF OZ

There is respectable strength, and then there is *aggression*. Please don't be confused by those with bigger personalities who insist they are "strong people." In my experience, they are anything but strong. These types are likely to interrupt your public dining experience with their loud monologues and raucous laughter. "That's enough about me. So, tell me . . . what do you think about me?" I refer to these characters as Wizard of Oz personalities. (Behind all of the steam, loud noises, and a terrifying mask, Dorothy found a scared little man—not the sort of person to instill confidence in others.) A revealing question to ask is, "Would you pass the tea bag test?" It's really hard to tell what sort of tea bag you have once they are out of the packets. You take two out, and head over to the two different cups, only to forget which is the licorice and which is the chamomile. You have a 50 percent chance of getting it right, so you place the bags in the cups and add boiling water. And there you have it. Let's hope you got it right! The story goes that people can present in largely the same way on the surface, and you don't really know what you've got until they are in a pressured situation (hot water).

## FEELING A LITTLE BIT RATTLED?

A lot longer ago than I care to remember I was told of a laboratory experiment involving physical stress responses in rats. I have found no written report to back this. Apparently a family of rats was divided into two groups and placed on opposite sides of a laboratory. They were given identical living conditions except for *environmental safety*. One group was handled gently with softly spoken care and attention; the others were subject to loud voices and rough treatment and had their cage rattled and banged every time someone passed by. The first group thrived, and the second group developed spotty rashes and began to lose their hair. The only difference between the two groups was the level of daily stress they were exposed to.

But the work of Dr. Hans Selye (born in 1907 in Vienna Hungary died in 1982 in Montreal Quebec)[2] was documented. Hanse is attributed to be the first to demonstrate the existence of biological stress.

Selye observed similar symptoms in patients with chronic illnesses like tuberculosis and cancer which he later tested on rodents. The symptoms he identified are now commonly known as the stress response. Selye identified three stress response phases, Resistance, Adaptation, and finally, Exhaustion, preceding death.

What sort of cellular leader are you? You govern your own trillions of cells, so take a moment to really think whether you are in fact a weak, tyrannical, and oppressive leader, or strong, considerate, and consultative. All thoughts and actions controlling your vitality are your responsibility. Every moment of every day, your body is controlled by your thoughts, actions, and stress levels. Are you their lion on the rock or their Wizard of Oz? Do you want your body to be overrun by anarchists? If you respond to any signal from your cellular community with anything less than love and care, you can expect revolt. By murdering your own subjects with alcohol or drugs, you give them no option but to riot and burn tires and vehicles in your streets. By persisting with junk food, exhaustion, stress, stinky thinking, shallow breathing, and lack of exercise, you force them into smashing your windows and setting your internal buildings alight to be heard. As long as they are ignored, they have no choice but to continue looting, rioting, and smashing you down from the inside in an attempt to get your attention. They will continue with this behavior until their concerns are not only received but resolved. Your body can't replace you with another leader. It is stuck with you and the decisions you make every day, healthy or unhealthy. If your symptoms, whatever they might be, are getting worse, you might want to spare a thought for all of the residents who make up *you*. The ones acting out through "dis-ease" are trying to get your attention.

## NEVER STOP!

All too often we distract ourselves from our internal alarm system by keeping busy. This mindset can take on a life of its own, morphing into a state of just "busy being busy." Once this way of life is instilled, any gap in our day can feel extremely uncomfortable. It's a way to "stop the sky from falling." We can become driven by self-perpetuating negative thoughts, knowing full well that if we were to rest, even for a moment, something terrible would happen.

*You can do a quick check of the current state of your own system now if you like. Just hold your hands out as still as you can in front of you. Any movement indicates a body desperate to move.*

If your body has been accustomed to hearing from you only when you have useful information for it to respond to, your hands, which reflect the state of your whole body, will be relaxed. When held parallel with the ground, the ends of your fingers will droop a little as they rest, awaiting your next command. Having learned to trust your strong, relaxed leadership, they will get used to only being called on when actually needed and will not twitch. On the other hand, any finger trembling or twitching gives you a visual reflection of a body in a state of unrest. If you have been rushing, obsessing, and worrying, you are probably not aware of the stream of useless information you have been sending out to *all* of the cells in your body. Imagine how you would feel if your neighbors kept knocking on your door every hour of every day to check on you. Just like the disturbed rats, any *body* under this constant disturbance from Wizard of Oz leadership will literally become dis-eased.

## THE MEDIA

As we sit still, the news presenter unflinchingly demonstrates to us that there is no need to react, even while introducing footage with, "Please be aware that some of the images you are about to see are graphic and may be disturbing." The Russian/Ukrainian and Israeli/Palestinian conflicts, with their steadily rising death tolls, are beamed into our lounges daily. Close-ups of carnage and dead bodies are flashed on the screen, many of them civilians, showcasing men, women, and children being slaughtered. The next featured news story is a major pile-up involving multiple fatalities on an American highway. Without batting an eyelid, a story about a rugby player and his new baby is detailed. Next are countless ads designed to deceive: "MUST END MONDAY! up to 50% OFF STOREWIDE. Terms and conditions apply. See in store for details." Then it's back to North Korea's leader, who has fired a missile over Japan into the ocean. Sources reveal he is planning a live nuclear test. That horror is followed by the latest weather-related disaster, a mudslide wiping out an entire village, killing thousands, and is thought to be linked to climate change. Then another advert, this time from a corporation inappropriately using the word *love*. And what do we do next? Our internal reply? *Shall I have sour cream and chives, or salt and vinegar chips tonight?*

In 1983 there was a nationwide reaction to a little girl's body being found on the beach at Napier. Kirsa Jenson had been horse riding alone and, once discovered dead, was presumed to have been abducted and murdered. It is a very sad case that is yet to be solved. This news sparked a nationwide shift. Overnight, parents began ferrying their children to and from school because suddenly it was no longer safe in New Zealand for kids to find their own way. But now in 2024, we have become reasonably comfortable with one or two murders every week. We are learning to internalize massive amounts of stress in our daily lives by *not reacting*. We all feel the tension building, but in most situations, we don't react anymore. Whether we stay still because we might be embarrassed to react, or we are fearful of being judged, or we think it's cool not to move, we become frozen. Our breathing becomes shallow and stifled, and our physical world steadily shrinks. If you don't use it, you lose it, and sitting still with our minds whizzing, somewhere in between a little rushed and terrified, teaches our bodies over and again not to react to anything. By continuing to stay physically frozen in time while being chemically prodded to leap around, we begin a slow death. I say *terrified, leap around*, and *slow death* because the request from our nervous system is never a small one. The origins of fight-or-flight are in life-or-death matters; internally, this is as big as anything ever gets. This involuntary shutting down could very well be the initiator of diseases like Parkinson's. Recent studies have proven that gross movement (large movements using the arms, legs, and torso), if done regularly, can slow or even halt the progress of this debilitating disease.[3] What if that is what has been missing? Another likely example is Tourette Syndrome. This involves not only involuntary movements but verbalizing as well. A body that is constantly shut down, unable to respond to any of this powerful repetitive stimulus, year after year, desperate to react, finally finds its own way through. Imagine if your chemical stress signals were replaced by a person whose job it was to poke, prod, and prompt you. Not just now and then; this would be going on most of the time, including when you are trying to sleep. These jabs would not be of the gentle kind. Delivered by a messenger from a life-and-death system, they would probably feel more like needles. How long, I wonder, could you stay silent? By adopting anything but a vibrant physical reaction, you are steadily losing your vitality.

We become so good at staying still while being chemically and electrically requested to respond that our nervous reactions begin to override our own perceived limitations. Movements begin to creep through. The next time you go to the mall, have a look around the food hall. Among those sitting and eating, there will be at least one or two with one of their legs nervously bouncing up and down.

This total lack of vitality in the presence of stimulation is responsible for a massive list of diseases. We are literally "stewing in our own juices." This potent mixture of tension toxins and total lack of response generates pain, the management of which is turning us into junkies. According to Medino Online,[4] in the UK alone an estimated 6,300 tons of paracetamol is sold annually. That's 35 tons per million. This equates to seventy tablets each per year. If you prefer a visual representation, that's 315 twenty-ton diggers.

What we all need to understand is the fact that it has always been up to us. It's our decision whether or not we buy into the "gerbil on the wheel" way of living that requires only a couple of pills to start or end each day. Nothing will ever change until we decide to do something different than we have always done by stepping off the treadmill. Real, lasting change requires us to engage in what I call the three selfs: *self-honesty, self-responsibility,* and *self-discipline.* There is space and time required to do any one thing properly and correctly to completion without risking injury. What we do over and over is try and distort this truth and attempt to prove this simple fact wrong until we're blue in the face. By taking on too much, forcing unrealistic deadlines, and rushing, we create our own pressure. Just take a look at any of the reality TV shows. More and more time pressure is applied to the contestants because we are entertained by their inevitable failure. We love to watch others pushed to the point of meltdown.

## CANCER

According to the World Health Organization Mortality Database 2020, 10 million deaths (one in six) were caused by cancer.[5] If anyone had asked me when I began to write this book if I would broach the subject of cancer, my answer would have been, "Never in a million years." But here, five years later I can confidently say that cancer must surely be the ultimate bodily manifestation of unrest. Body cells want to help us, and when they are calmly and clearly directed, they do just that. But when compacted and highly inflamed, then subject to a relentless stream of nonspecific demands from a mind that is feeling powerless and desperately unsettled, they don't know what to do. Persistent negative thoughts must surely cause the most self-destructive internal confusion: *I want change but I have no idea what I really want or how to achieve any of it. I've been so upset for so long, and I really want things to be different from the way that they are.* Any person not feeling good enough or unsatisfied in any way will transfer that powerful self-destructive message down their internal chain of command so strongly and so often that their cells will attempt to accommodate their leader by manifesting changes. In an attempt to satisfy the repetitive nonspecific requests for things to be different, abnormal cells are built. These groupings of cells are usually faulty and what we collectively recognize as cancer. With the initial job done and the signals of unrest still coming through strongly, the cells will try to further their helping response by beginning a process of migration called metastasizing. In this process, the faulty cells move to other parts of the body where they set up camp and go about making more *improvements.*

In relation to this, I have been tracking the locations of body tensions in men with cancer diagnoses. All of those diagnosed with either chronic inflammatory groin pain, severely elevated PSA, or prostate cancer diagnosis presented at their initial appointment with locked sacroiliac joints, completely immobilizing the sacrum. All of those presenting with testicular inflammation or testicular cancer diagnosis presented with painfully compressed and misaligned L2, L3, and L4 (center of the lower back). It makes sense to consider the possibility of projecting this same scenario of cause and effect to other regions of the body, such as the base of the neck and cancers of the mouth and throat, or mid thoracic affecting the upper gastric region.

Please forgive me for this awful example, but our current fearful, pressured existence presents the same scenario for our bodies as if you were to lock yourself in the garage, open the car windows, and rev the engine. The steadily building toxins would eventually kill you; likewise, so will this ridiculous, unrested way of living. Maybe not all at once, but slowly and surely it is lethal. If you can help to rid the world of the carnage that is constantly available to us through the media, then great. But for the rest of us, it is important to stay informed up to a point and then use what all electronic devices have: the off switch.

## CHAPTER 6

# REINVIGORATION

## COMMON LANGUAGE

*"Comfortable in my own skin."*
*"A rolling stone gathers no moss."*
*"I'm a bit of a perfectionist."*

## QUICK FIX

Healthy living requires harmony between mind and body speeds. It's a lot easier to move the body than to slow our busy brains, so get a minimum of a half hour, three times every week, of aerobic activity to make you puff, synchronizing your body with your busy mind.

Engineering design prevents us from ruining our cars. Enough engines have been destroyed in controlled situations to establish their safe operating limits. I'm not sure if this is still done today, but they used to bolt fully assembled new motors into test beds and rev them continuously until they blew up. This "rev it until it blows up" testing produced the data required to establish the point where shifting up to the next gear would lower the revolutions per minute (rpm) to a safe level. This gear shift reduces the revs until the car moves more. But how do we apply this to ourselves, and how do we know where our red line is? I'm sure anyone who has burned themselves out would advise you against blowing your own engine to find out. This massive disconnect we have built between our mind and body desperately needs reconciliation.

## EDNA'S CAR

Many years ago, there was a retired widow who owned a mint-green Morris 1100. Once a week, Edna drove the half mile from her home to park in the center of town outside the club. From there, she could pull her two-wheeled tartan trolley bag to the dairy, T.A.B, general store, or hairdresser. Then she would go into the club for a shandie (a mix of beer and lemonade) before driving home. The car never got up to running temperature, which choked it up and gave it a telltale sooty tailpipe. Once a year, always in spring, she would bring it to her mechanic, telling him that it wasn't driving very well, and asked if he could fix it. The answer was always the same. "No problem, Edna. Just leave it with me. I'll have it ready for you this afternoon." He knew that all of the short-tripping at low speed had clogged it up again, and all that was needed was a good "blow-out." With Edna safely out of view, off he went on a fast trip that would last about forty-five minutes. He'd drive up one side of the river valley, go across the bridge, then down the other side, and back to the garage. Most of the way up the valley it coughed and spluttered; low on power it left a swirling trail of blue haze out the back. Through lack of use, the wheel cylinders were stuck, which made the brakes dangerously ineffective. At about the halfway point, everything started to improve. The brakes became more responsive, the power about doubled, and the dull spiraling haze that had followed him up the valley was gone, restoring the gunmetal gray tailpipe characteristic of a healthy engine. Edna, having no idea what had just happened, paid the very modest bill and drove her "repaired car" back home. As she drove away, she could tell in an instant that it was running so much better and probably thought what a clever man he was to be able to fix all of those faults in such a short time.

You can't imagine Edna sitting in her motionless car, revving the engine for hours on end, but that is exactly what we are doing with our bodies. Deterioration resulting from underutilization is bad enough on its own, but then we exacerbate our situation. Rushing to achieve deadlines, we sit mismatched, enslaved to our electronic devices, our bodies sedentary, hunched over with our brain climbing mountains. By continuing to be nonresponsive in the face of a relentless onslaught of irrational fear-based stimulation, we become saturated with stress hormones that are both choking and stifling us. The most extreme example of this is online gaming. The mind and body could not be more separated than while sitting, moving only our thumbs as we run, hide, stalk, and shoot "virtual" beings in endless kill-or-be-killed scenarios! Over time, this pattern becomes so entrenched that the body alarms become barely registerable. I imagine the "react" body voice mentioned earlier walking away, leaving the stress response taps wide open and the brain's "no" eventually becoming something more like a "yeah, whatever." We are in trouble once this contemptuous mind-body communication gap is created.

## CHAOS

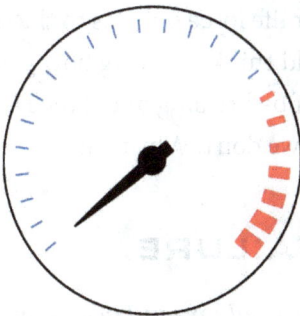 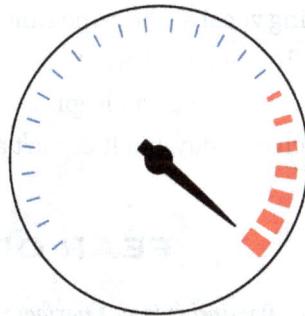

## BODY        MIND

## SELF-CONSCIOUSNESS

Being conscious of ourselves is a major problem, and it is only possible when we are in our heads. This is one of our most common barriers to synchronizing mind and body speeds. The anxiety generated by self-consciousness stops us from automatically transitioning into the safe zone? For thousands of years the world over, indigenous peoples have been bridging the gap between mind and body by dancing and singing. It usually begins with a small rhythmic group. Inevitably, the infectious rhythms rapidly spread to involve the whole village in a sea of voices, movement, and celebration that lasts for hours. If you have ever been a tourist entertained by one of these groups, you will have felt the difference. Most onlookers sit rigidly, all the while surrounded by exuberance, frozen in collective discomfort. It's not really all that surprising coming from a background of spiritual celebration being limited to standing motionless in rows between church pews, singing about love, creation, and joy. Charismatic churchgoers have been singing and moving for years; they all know that it literally lifts spirits. Revitalization is essential for good mind and body health. This is not new information. Most of us already know the mental and physical health benefits of regular movement, but when this is coupled with becoming vocal at the same time, our life force bubbles to the surface and we become exuberant! You would think knowing how good this feels would have us all leaping out of bed to sing and dance our way into each new day, but it doesn't and we don't. Why is that?

## FEAR OF FAILURE

*What if I try and it is not perfect? That would mean I'm a failure, and I just couldn't stand that.* But if you don't try you have already failed. Japanese ceramic artists at the top of their game apparently always leave a tiny flaw. This is to dissolve the pressure of perfectionism. The pieces that they create are some of the best in the world. Without the very closest scrutiny, their intentional flaw would go undetected. Throughout the whole process, the person creating each piece is able to relax in the knowledge that they have, in their intentional failure, already succeeded. They have removed the temptation to pressurize themselves by striving for the unachievable. In this relaxed state, and with the absence of performance anxiety, their creative juices are allowed to flow freely, greatly enhancing their ability to create. Encountering failure on your road to any success is inevitable. You can easily find motivational quotes from successful people who have *failed* multiple times. There is another Japanese ceramic art called *kintsugi* where broken, usually vessels, are repaired using gold-dusted urushi. Rather than trying to hide the flaws this method highlights the damage in celebration of the history it represents. This method teaches us that in life we can turn adversity into something that is beautiful and resilient.

## AVOIDING AVOIDANCE

A good start on the road to mental and physical freedom is to stop telling yourself little white lies. If any part of your life is out of control and the situation is having a negative impact on you, the way to avoid change is to tell yourself that it is not your doing. By convincing yourself that any situation is someone else's fault, you avoid self-responsibility. Until you can accept that you are the only one who can implement the changes you need to make, there is no hope of you having any influence over outcomes. This denial can put you on a slippery slope on the edge of a black hole to self-destruction. Being honest with yourself makes room for hope. Incorporating self-honesty into any situation sounds like this: "I realize this situation is causing me harm, but up until now I have been choosing to do nothing about it."

Taking this leap opens the door to that voice deep inside yourself that says, *What you are currently doing is unhealthy.* Whether you pay attention to it or not, it has always been there. Listening to it once is a good start, but in order to succeed you will need to keep this line of communication open. A few silent minutes set aside each day to tune into your internal alarm system is a good place to begin. Soon, you may encounter another very effective avoidance strategy: having a high pain tolerance.

## HIGH PAIN TOLERANCE

"Oh, I'm okay. I can just keep going. I've got a really high pain tolerance." This is a learned coping mechanism that has to be unlearned in order to succeed. Usually, it is the result of being in pain for a long time. All it means is that you have become really good at ignoring your internal alarm system. The failure of body parts or systems whose alarms are chronically overridden is inevitable. Unanswered pain signals inevitably lead to eventual localized breakdowns. This level of incremental ignorance is a bit like suddenly relocating under the flight path of a busy airport. At first the noise would drive you mad. But give it a year or so, and when asked by your visitors, "How can you stand the noise from all of those planes?" you will answer, "Planes? What planes?" As you reinstate pain receptive awareness, you may begin to notice a few body signals that you were not even aware of. A bit like the rattling sounds we heard in our cars, we were only aware of the loudest one.

### PETER

*"Thank you. My hip is feeling much better. I think you must have done something to my shoulder, though, because it has started to really hurt. It was okay before you began working on me." Peter did not have any new pain. He simply began to feel the lower intensity pains once the more acute pain signals subsided. (As his perception improved, he began to hear all of the "planes" again.) Once Peter successfully tuned in to receiving the more subtle distress signals sent to him, his body made the shift*

*into feeling heard. Experiencing his more empathetic, responsive leader-*
*ship restored order among all of his cellular residents, who ceased pro-*
*testing and went back to maintaining health and harmony. So how do we*
*make the shift into harmonious mind-body existence?*

If you are experiencing this internal separation with your mind
revving high and running amok, and your body is feeling resigned to
a life of defeat, you will need to close the gap. You have two choices
here; you can either reduce the speed of your mind or move your body
more. If your day job was hunting dinosaurs to feed your family, you
would be active enough to avoid this problem. Even if you did lie awake
at night, your body riddled with stress hormones, wondering if you
would be mauled or eaten at the next hunt, the physical exertion
required to kill one of those giants with a sharp stone on a stick would
more than balance out any mind-body distancing. For most people,
the option of slowing the mind is the more difficult one. In our current
version of reality, instant gratification has reached epidemic proportions. Any attempt to harness our minds that whiz around like a ger-
bil-powered wheel seems to most of us insurmountable. If you can't
slow that racing one down, you have to speed up the sluggish one, so
moving your body becomes the obvious choice. I'm not suggesting
that you do this all at one go like the mechanic did for Edna's car. That
would be risking injury. But if your body is clogged and unresponsive
from relative underutilization, then you need *reinvigoration*. What we
can do for ourselves is roll up our metaphorical garage door and take
our body out for a spin.

## THE PAIN OF GAIN

Edana's car did not suddenly leap back to full potential and neither
can we. Her mechanic needed to struggle her car most of the way up
one side of the river valley before performance and braking began to
improve. This is what to expect from your body once you decide to
re-invigorate. Once you have begun any restorative exercise program

you will notice straight away that your breathing is labored and the next day your muscles will be a bit sore. All this means is that you are pushing hard enough up against the point to which your body has deteriorated. The answer is very simple, keep going. Within recommended limits doing a little bit often will gradually restore your full potential to breathe and move. Dr. Michael Mosley[1] is worth looking up. He has done several documentaries on body rejuvenation through diet and exercise.

## PETER

*A strapping young chap in the prime of his life, Peter had suffered a very serious motor vehicle accident, and after two years of conventional treatment, he was still struggling with what he described as "daily agony." He had been told that all recovery options had been exhausted; therefore, pain management was now his only option. He appeared at my clinic after being shoulder tapped by one of my existing clients, who suggested, "Why not go and see my guy? He fixed me." Following a block of initial twice-weekly sessions, Peter was feeling consistently better and confidently reduced his visits to my clinic down to fortnightly, then once every month. Sometime later, there was a bit of mystery around why he was regressing. Curious to know what had caused the setback, I asked him about his lifestyle. It turned out that Peter had no downtime. He was either working or asleep. Or, more accurately, he was trying to sleep. Once we established that stress was what had caused him to regress, I suggested he begin aerobic exercise in the form of a thirty-minute run three times a week. Peter returned a month later, ecstatic, informing me that he was back to his old self again and no longer required any remedial sessions. He brought the speed of his body up to the speed of his mind and, seemingly miraculously, released himself from pain.*

Do something aerobic every week to bring your body speed up to that of your mind. This regular exercise needs to be intense enough and often enough to flush out the toxins as they build. There is no

# HARMONY

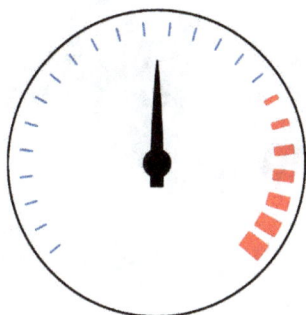 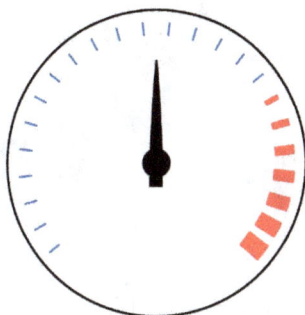

BODY    MIND

hard-and-fast rule for which exercise works the best or how much is the right amount. Simply set the pace to your own ability. Aim for at least half an hour three times every week of aerobic activities that make you puff a little. Choose an exercise like walking, jogging, rowing, cycling, swimming, or dancing, and you will be on the right track.

Oh, I nearly forgot. There is one more common obstacle. You can't jump-start anyone else's car unless your own battery is fully charged. Before you say you have no time for self-care because you need to look after your wife, your husband, your parents, your pets, your children, or your work commitments, let the martyr behavior go. You can look after everyone else so much better if you are in your best possible condition. That means being rested, nourished, exercised, and stretched.

There, it feels a lot better with that *off my chest*! Now on with what we inherit.

# CHAPTER 7

# BORN BEHIND THE EIGHT BALL

## COMMON LANGUAGE

*"Of course my son will play footy. It's in his blood."*
*"It's second nature."*
*"Chip off the old block."*

## QUICK FIX

Our human Internal Operating System is transferred via living tissue at conception. This behavior bank, modified experientially through the centuries, dictates our individual preferred perspective, language, thought processing, and behavior. Reprogramming is possible, albeit laborious. Repeating positive behaviors moves them to your home screen where they are more readily available, making them easier to repeat. Always start with a very subtle shift. Begin by looking in the mirror daily and saying, "I really like you, [state your name]."

All that we are physically as a newborn baby entering this world comes directly from our parents' genes, the rest we learn as we grow, or does it? I remember my father's voice here, who was known for his cutting one-liners: "In order to be healthy, choose your parents wisely."

The popular misconception seems to be that we are each born as a brand-spanking-new human being, like a photocopied image produced onto a clean new page. Just take the genes of two people, mix them up, and produce a totally new image. But are you in fact new, separate, and individual? It took me a long time to get my head around this next seemingly simple concept because my mind prefers to distance myself from a personal gene pool fraught with challenges; however, *you are not a copy only bearing a resemblance to your ancestors. You continued previous lives as two living cells. Both are alive, one given to you from each of your biological parents.*[1]

Two living cells from two individuals amalgamate, multiply, and grow. This is a combined continuation rather than a brand-new, isolated beginning. Neither the DNA nor the container die in this process. A tiny piece taken from a tree can be grown into a new tree that will stand long after the original has passed. So it is with us. As a new being, a living mixture of everything your parents were, did, and believed transferred to you at the moment of your conception. This tissue has been continuously alive, passing from person to person since the beginning of our existence.

We like to think that we are new, individual, unique, and totally unprogrammed. A blank slate onto which we can carve any life we choose. One where all of our decisions, actions, and reactions are our own, independent, and original. The reality, though, is that our thought processes are chosen, repeated, and modified by all of those who came before us. During pregnancy, thanks to the shared blood supply, each pre-birth baby's immune system receives some valuable programming from its mother's blood, but other than that, little more than sustenance is introduced. So, what do we really inherit? Genetics take care of how we look, such as the color of our eyes and hair, our skin type, and our stature. Predisposition toward health conditions is also in the mix, but what else crosses over? Language, likes, dislikes, prejudice, behavior, and preferences as well as experiences, habits, and beliefs are all inherited.

## "YOU'RE A CHIP OFF THE OLD BLOCK!"

We have a multitude of mannerisms, and each client I see is different. That is, unless they are a child of an existing client. They display, without exception, the actions, phrases, and mannerisms matching their parents, like a "minnie me." This is most obvious in their greetings and departures. There have been plenty of instances where I have heard people talking like their parents. Even though we swear that "we will never talk to our children like that," we do. You can well imagine that if we hear something said to us over and over as children, it can easily become ingrained in our heads. But what if that's not the case?

I had been friends with a couple who I used to visit for coffee and a chat on a fairly regular basis. This was, for the most part, an enjoyable experience for all concerned. Except for the way in which the man greeted my dog. He spoke in a voice he'd use while talking to baby: "Aww! Who's a little coochada woochada?" It was said with the same particularly silly accent every time, jarring my brain!

This couple eventually separated, and sometime later the ex-wife informed me that when they were teenagers, they had an unplanned baby. Their baby boy had been taken away for adoption at the hospital so soon after birth that he saw his mother once and never got to meet his father. Thirty-five years later she had been able to locate their son, now an adult with children of his own, and had arranged to meet him at the local airport. The mother and son called in to see me for an introductory visit before the long drive up the coast where he could meet his dad for the first time. They had not been in my home for more than a minute when my dog walked in. My jaw must have dropped to the floor when, seeing my dog, the son said the same phrase: "Aww! Who's a little coochada woochada?" Not only did he say the same words, but he said them in exactly the same nauseating way!

Since then, I have become increasingly interested in people's accounts *in a similar vein*, like the woman who received a handwritten letter from her biological father, wishing to meet her. He was reaching out to let her know how he had eventually found her and then asked if she would like to meet. His handwriting was identical to hers. Another person, who had yet to meet his biological parent, appeared to be a pea from the same pod as his estranged father. I quote, "He looked the same, had the same laugh, mannerisms, manner of speech, sense of humor, sentence phrasing, and intonation. He spoke with the same authority and had the same interests in aviation and broadcasting."

Well recognized is the fact that if you want to buy a dog that doesn't have a mean streak, you had better stick to reputable breeders. Why? Because they systematically eliminate undesirable personality and physical traits. How does this apply to humans? You have probably come across a few people who quite naturally err more toward snarling and biting your hand than smiling and shaking it gently. Before I attempt to explain how I believe this behavior is inherited, another example can be found in birds.

## BIRDS & BEHAVIOR

Birds build nests, lots of them! They masterfully create hundreds of different designs, each specific to their own species. Swallows create mud-spit balls and glue them together to form a pouch barely big enough to hold their growing chicks. Starlings, locating an access hole into a ceiling, build their nest by throwing straw into a massive heap. Then there are the weavers. Using around 1,000 supple grasses, they weave a hanging basket with an access hole in the side. My personal favorite has to be the red oven bird. Once the weather is wet enough, they use freshly formed mud mixed with tiny bits of straw and build something that closely resembles a pizza oven on top of a fence post. The opening, just big enough, is always constructed on the side facing away from the prevailing weather. Incredibly, they also add an

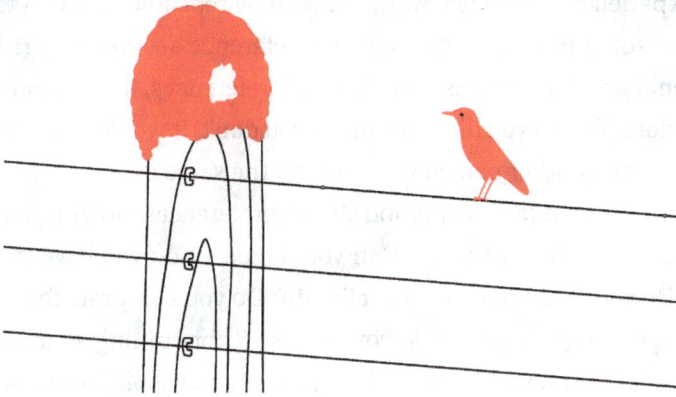

internal wall with an elevated access hole to the back room. This provides an added level of security against predators. With no plans to work from, they build the whole thing the same way that their parents did. Why has a starling never thought, *What the hell? Should I build one of those red oven bird nests this year? They look super cool, and I won't have to search for a roof with a hole in it to fill with straw.*

While young birds are growing toward adulthood, they never once see the completed nest, its shape, or how it was constructed. Yet they replicate it perfectly a year later. Birds must inherit a complete set of nest-building instructions, including not only the plans but the methods. Even more remarkable are the lyrebirds. The male builds a staging area on which to dance, and the female constructs the nest in a separate location, a dual process repeated through the generations. The male chicks do not see the stage or the dance, yet they repeat the process over and over.

It's been well-documented that we have both conscious and subconscious minds. It must be the subconscious part that carries this information, operating more like a reference section. Without any ability to discern or decide anything, the subconscious mind simply records and makes the information available to the conscious mind. A place to work *from* rather than *in*. This time bank, passed on from parents to children since the beginning of time, contains countless life experiences compiled away, ready to be repeated. You can take a look at some of what is in your own reference section by writing a personal list of your likes and dislikes, preferences, habits, and go-to behaviors. Things you like and things you don't. It would be extremely rare to find another person with exactly the same list.

Color, music, food, wine, and cheese preferences. How do you have your coffee or tea or herbal? Can you dance, or do you have two left feet? Do you prefer a hot or cold climate? Do you enjoy rain for the life it brings to the planet, or do you despise it for ruining your outside activity? What about singing? Can you sing like a bird, are you tone deaf, or do you land somewhere in between? Do you have a green thumb? Are you patient or not? Are you passive or aggressive, loud or quiet, cruisy or edgy? Fears are another great revealer. There are so many to choose from: spiders, snakes, deep water, scorpions, dogs, heights, open spaces, public speaking, tight spaces, the dark, being alone, crowded spaces, the outdoors, the sea, flying, diving, boating, people? Your personality is probably better filled out by someone else. Our self-image is always tainted with misconceptions. To get a better understanding of your inherited personality traits, video yourself. This is your chance to see yourself how others see you.

*Simply prop your phone up where the camera can take in the whole room, with their permission of course. Record yourself interacting with others for at least ten minutes. You will see in an instant that your actions and reactions are individual.*

I witnessed a striking example of the difference in our thinking patterns years ago while attending a redundancy meeting. In a room of about forty employees, we all heard the same speech about our impending incremental doom from the CEO. Some left the room, joking about what they would have for morning tea, while one left in tears and never returned. He suffered a total breakdown.

Every person's life is experienced through their own interpretation of it. How else could we be so different from one another? What else could make you the class clown or the quiet child, and why can't we switch roles? In the same way as a starling never builds an oven bird nest, we are all pre-programmed by what our parents and their parents inherited, experienced, and did most often. I'm told that if a self-made rich and poor person are switched, they rapidly revert back to their previous ways because they don't know how to be any different than they are. What records this huge historical databank in a way that it can be passed on? The answer is surprisingly simple. We all have an *internal operating system.*

## INTERNAL OPERATING SYSTEM (IOS)

Let's refer back to the birds. The only way for birds to have inherited their unique behavioral preferences is through an already pro-grammed operating system. I know, having read Bill Bryson's fasci-nating book, *A Short History of Nearly Everything,*[2] that the information stored in our DNA is huge, but it doesn't have the capacity to do all of that. There is a transfer of programming. There is no other logical way to explain the birds being able to build their own particular species-specific nests, or the dogs responding to situations in the same way that their unseen parents have.

If you look inside a mobile phone using a microscope, you will never find the IOS, and it's the same for our own personal system. Neither can be seen. Living tissue carrying each individual's IOS has been transferring across the invisible databank to each new being since the beginning of time. Those of us alive now are unconsciously carrying around in our collective subconscious minds the complete history of the human race. Not just whatever happened in our parents' lives, but the entire ancestral line, right across time. You don't have to watch too many historical dramas on television to get an understand-ing of why we still struggle as a species. Our history is full of blood-thirsty violence, chaos, and dishonesty, even cannibalism. We have been murdering each other in wars, using capital punishment, and ripping each other off all through the ages. Is it any wonder we have trouble changing our behavior? Being overlaid so many times must surely make it the proverbially well-worn path.

## MARY

*"My neck has stiffened up so much that I can no longer turn my head. The specialist said I have a nerve pinched somewhere. I'm getting migraines again and can't sleep. It's even going down my arm. I have to lie on two pillows and get the angle of my head just right to ease the nerve pain. I feel terrible. What's causing all of this?"*

*"Same as it has always been, Mary," I said. "It's just a buildup of stress in your body. You really need regular sessions to keep on top of it. Or you could learn to slow down."*

*"I need to stop? Good luck with that."*

*We booked six sessions over the first three weeks and then two more per week after that, both knowing full well that once the pain levels were consistently less than a four out of ten, she would cancel the rest of the appointments, only to return a year later asking the same question again. Mary's programming was preventing her from taking her recovery any further than the bare minimum.*

# WE GET GOOD AT WHAT WE DO EVERY DAY

It's incredibly hard to change something that has been programmed for centuries. But it can be done. To act in a different way (just like a bird building a different nest), we not only have to find, download, and install a different program, we have to operate it often enough to move it to the home screen and keep it there. As with any IOS, there are many screens with which to interact, but it is this home screen that contains all of our most commonly used applications. We don't choose what gets programmed into these apps on our inherited list. Imagine if we could sit down and decide our behavioral traits.

*"Let's see now . . . I need to download a new program that will kill a lot of birds all with the same stone. There it is, with the title 'Stay calm, no matter what's going on.' It must surely go a long way toward improving my mental and physical health. Far out! Do they really expect me to pay that much for it? Not only is it breathtakingly expensive, but I have to use it every day or it evaporates. And then I have to buy it all over again Seriously? Oh well. If it fixes the problem, I guess I'll just have to put it on the mortgage or pay it off on my credit card."*

Getting back to the chapter's title, Born Behind the Eight Ball, this is the single most difficult position to play from in a game of snooker. If either your mother or father is managing life anxiously and reactively, you have about a fifty-fifty chance of inheriting the same settings. If both of your parents behave this way, it is possible to receive a double whammy. Anxious and reactive plus anxious and reactive combine to produce a very anxious and very reactive child. If this is the case for you, then your mind and your body will be perpetually inflamed. You will stress and worry constantly about the smallest of things, and your body will respond with inflammatory diseases both inside and out. Your fears, although very real to you, will be comparatively irrational, and you will constantly worry about something, rapidly replacing any resolved issue with a new unresolved one in what Peter calls "crisis de jour" (crisis of the day). Your body will accumulate and hold tension. You will tend to talk quickly, over others, and at length, and are often still talking when the subject has been exhausted. Your eyes will tend to dart around, and you will blink often while breathing in teaspoons of air. Your whole body will overreact to stimulus. It's not your fault; you don't get to choose any of this programming. The children I have treated over nearly three decades all share their individual holding patterns with their parents. Whether it's a few jammed ribs on the upper right side, or left lower back pain affecting the knee and ankle of the opposite side, all of their "knotty sore bits" can be found in their parents' bodies too.

## MARY

*In her eighties, she reminisced during a hip flexor release session about how it was normal to be beaten with a leather strap as a child at school and again at home, usually with a belt, on a regular basis.*

*"It was quite often not my fault. I was terrified and would have to hide under the bed or outside."*

Mary's home screen would have been dominated by apps relating to violence, fear, suffering, becoming invisible, and trying to stay safe. Beatings at home and school were commonplace at that time, and her fear-filled programming would have been overlaid many times before being passed to her offspring. Mary's children, inheriting her programming, would have wondered why they experienced difficulty interacting with others. We can only play with the cards we have been dealt. An inherited IOS double whammy of reactivity and anxiety places us on a daily operational set point above the inflammatory red line. So, what is this red line anyway? And what really happens if you move above it?

## CHAPTER 8

# LIFE ABOVE
# THE RED LINE

## COMMON LANGUAGE

*"I'm a bundle of nerves."*
*"I'm a nervous wreck."*
*"Such a busy body."*

## QUICK FIX

We either visit or at worst live above the red line where our fight-or-flight tendencies engage. Microbreaks, breath awareness, and learning to *rush slowly* all assist our return.

How many of our worries actually come true? A study with results published in 2019 by Noa Kegamaya, PhD revealed that on average, 91.39 percent of participants' worries did not come true. Only 8.61 percent of their worries did come true. For one out of every four, none of their worries came true. Which means for us that most of the time, our fears are unfounded.[1] Once we drift above the red line, we enter a space where things are no longer real. On a scale of one to ten, one being totally chilled and ten being worried constantly, there is a red line at around seven where symptoms, particularly skin reddening, appear. People at a one on this scale, after

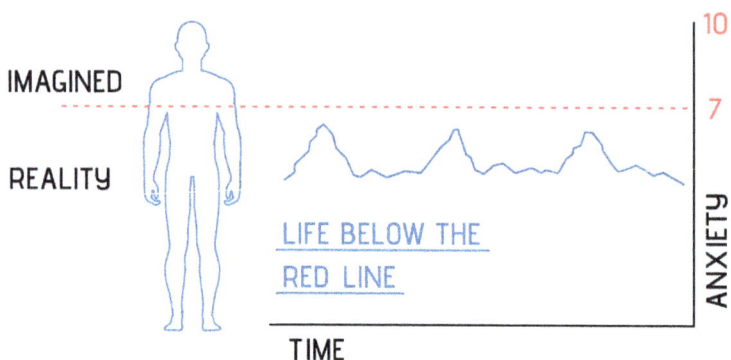

checking that everyone was safely outside their fully insured home, would calmly watch their house burning to the ground. Those at a ten are likely to smell the toast burning and run outside, adamant that the house is burning down. There is no chance of inner peace in the red zone. The whole body is in a perpetual state of high alert where the slightest irritant will trigger an overreaction. This is also the range where whatever we are genetically predisposed to is able to materialize. The only way to find good health and a relaxed state of mind is to adopt the habit of breathing yourself further down the scale.

Below the red line, we are connected to what is actually happening. We have our senses intact and receive unhampered signals from sight, sound, smell, taste, and touch. Our breathing includes the whole body, keeping us connected to each new moment as it unfolds. Our brain, fully functional, receives real-time messages, making decisions based on what is actually happening.

Once we go above the red line, our fight-or-flight instincts are triggered and our senses are reduced or overridden. Devoid of reliable sensory input, our brain is forced to decide what to do based on its own thoughts. The brain's ability to rationalize is further hampered by our survival mode having shut down some of its parts. Responding to the reality removing upward breath (inhaling up toward the neck), it is free to MSU (*make shit up*).

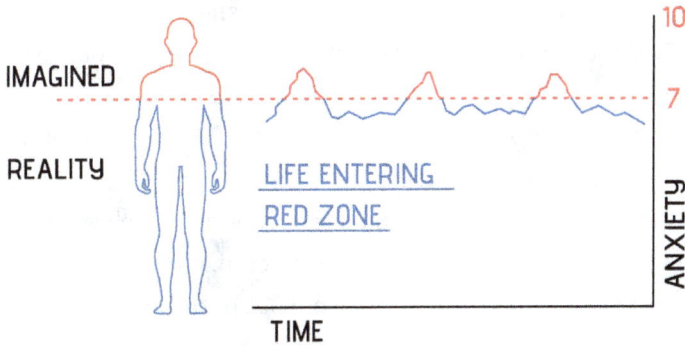

Witnessing something scary can take us momentarily above the line where we could develop and overlay a fear of whatever scared us. Because it's only a blip of seven on the scale, the fear does not get trapped. Experiencing the difference between above and below the line makes it possible for us to compare the two states: scared and not scared. It's a completely different story for those of us who have inherited a daily reality of living above seven. In this position, fear is part of everyday life. Body awareness and breathing all reside in the chest, neck, and head. This existence ensures that we are constantly frazzled.

## "I FEEL A BIT FRAZZLED!"

The crippling reality for those who live totally above the red line is the fact that they have never experienced true relaxation. They experience

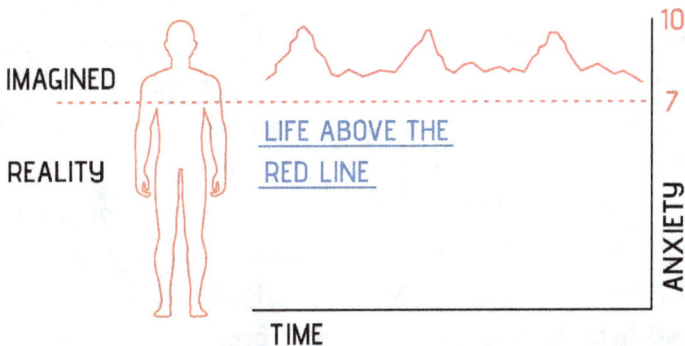

the same daily ups and downs, but the difference is that it all happens exclusively above seven. It's like the same window is mounted much higher on the wall. Their whole life experience is one of varying degrees of heightened intensity. Their totally relaxed 7.5 state is another person's "just got a fairly big fright" 7.5. It's a bit the same as asking a goldfish what water is. If they could talk, they would tell you that they have no idea. The only way for them to recognize water actually exists is through the lack of it by lifting them out of the bowl. It's the same with living above seven. There is no way to recognize the existence of anything less than a seven outside of actually having that experience. So, on about the tenth day at a tropical retreat with all the bells and whistles to assist relaxation, it can happen. Possibly for the first time ever, the person gets off the relaxing massage table, after a one-hour, zero-input flotation tank before the massage, and experiences *feeling something less than seven . . . a 6.9 perhaps?*

## MARY

*"I've been going to this new breathing coach. She is amazing! She is teaching me to slow down by breathing down into my body. It's really working, and when I use it, I feel more relaxed. What is incredible is that my memory is coming back. I have been forgetting things lately, and trying really hard to remember them does not work. Every time I practice the slow breathing exercise, I remember things again. It's just like magic!"*

The occupiers of the Bodies on the next page experience their *normal* lives differently. The one on the right lives above seven, in a state of permanent unrested inflammation. The one on the left does not live in a heightened state. Life in the inherited red zone tends to be difficult. With a body and mind that are normally inflamed, stress management is a daily necessity. I hasten to add that once identified, there are some excellent management tools that can be adapted to make a positive difference. Mary shared with me her pathway to recovery in the hope that it might help others:

NORMAL NORMAL

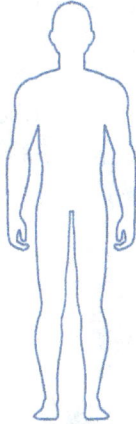 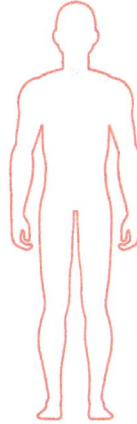

*"I have been in so much pain for such a long time and thought that it was all my fault. My default was to keep beating myself up. Firstly, for constantly feeling so bad. Secondly, for never being able to find a quick fix. It felt unfair that this kept happening to me. I needed to know that I was not crazy and that I hadn't imagined it. I got sick of being told that it was all in my head. All that ever did was make me feel worse and more out of control. Finally, I got it. What I needed to understand was the fact that we all have inherited weaknesses, and this particular one was mine. I wasn't crazy. None of this was my fault, and there is no quick fix; there never was. Understanding the fact that management was my only option allowed me to cut the crap and take responsibility for managing my own health by deciding on and fully committing to an appropriate self-maintenance program."*

## WIERDLY CALM

Mary at about session three began to understand how her daily existence above the red line had affected her whole body. Beginning to feel the difference between tense and a little more relaxed, Mary wondered why she had felt "weirdly calm" in a recent crisis situation. The Christchurch mosque shootings where 51 people were killed and another 89 injured by a lone gunman happened close to where she worked. Panic spread rapidly through the staff and Mary now wondered why herself, being such a nervous person, had been the one taking care of the others. Because Mary's daily existence was close to the top of the scale, her shift to ten out of ten took her up somewhere near two points. Any of the other more relaxed staff members who went to the same ten out of ten rocketed through a massive shift of somewhere near seven points!

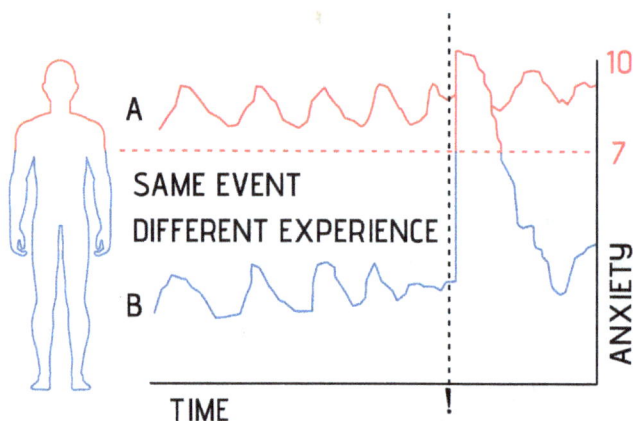

Daily anxiety levels can be reduced by choosing what we think. According to Dr. Fred Luskin a senior consultant in health promotion at Stanford University, we have somewhere near 60,000 thoughts every day, 90 percent of which are repetitive throughout the day and from the previous days.[2] If we tell ourselves over and over again throughout the day that something is not possible, or is scary, then it becomes a self-fulfilling prophecy. Getting good at what we do every day in a more positive direction entrenches lower levels of stress and anxiety. With any anxiety comes a feeling of urgency; therefore, in order to succeed, we need to select a level of repetitive change that is microscopic so as not to introduce any pressure. Doing even the tiniest bit in a positive direction each day flies in the face of the well-worn path of self-perpetuating failure, proving to ourselves that if we can succeed at one thing, however small, then maybe we can succeed at many things.

*Peter once came out with what I think is an absolute pearl. He said that the key is to "rush slowly," and maybe it is that simple. We can begin to harness those tens of thousands of daily thoughts once we decide to pull back, even just a little.*

## START BY STOPPING
## A LITTLE EVERY DAY

If we can pull back from the instant gratification for even a few seconds, we can remove a tiny spec of tension. By introducing infinitesimally small gaps, we begin to wear a new path. Even if we are only able to shift our compass bearing 0.01 degrees, we still take on a new course. Which means we eventually arrive at a different destination. So, how do we do it? It's as simple as taking a breath. You can't

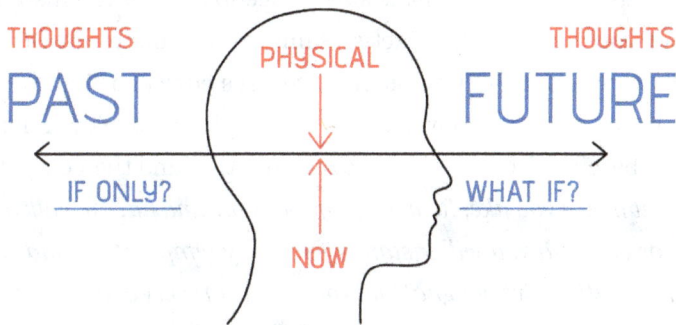

breathe in tomorrow, yesterday, or even a nanosecond forward or backward. Tuning into our breathing disengages us from all of the phantasmagorical thinking that is the red zone and returns us to our bodies. Another thing that brings us back to the present moment is any sudden flood of input from our senses. This is one of the reasons why it is so relaxing to smell the fragrance of a flower or eat something delicious. Both of these acts provide us with real-time input. The standout when it comes to returning to the moment has to be the recently popularized cold shower or even the ice bath. I challenge you to stand under a cold shower and worry. You simply cannot go forward or backward in your thinking with the tsunami of present-moment input that amount of cold sensation generates. A milder but still very effective way to reset during the day is to hold your hands under cold running water and then slap a little on your face or the back of your neck. Another is to walk barefoot. Last popularized in the late sixties and early seventies by the free-thinking hippies, this recent rediscovery is poised to be the next big thing in health-enhancing habits. It is sure to be attached to wonder filled claims of the life-giving miracles that occur once you tune your feet into the lay lines and energy fields that are generated by the earth. That may well be so, and you can be sure that health retreats will tap into selling that concept. But on a purely basic body system level, walking in barefeet is simply calming your mind by keeping you present. It's what we call *being brought back down to earth.* As long as you wear your shoes and socks, your feet are kept at a fairly even temperature and you get very little surface feedback. But the instant you stand on your bare feet, feedback streams toward your brain. Of course, the ultimate source of input is in the water's edge of a slightly grainy sandy beach on a cold day. But you can begin in your own home by walking barefoot from a wooden deck onto tiles and then carpet.

*Try it now if you like. Remove your footwear and have a walk around inside or out, and you will instantly feel every temperature and surface texture variation. Every signal that you receive in every changing moment helps to keep you in your body rather than your head!*

In my decades of practice, no one has ever noticed that before I process any transaction on my debit/credit machine, I take in a gentle breath and pause for three seconds as I let it go. These are some of my daily micropauses. I say confidently that no one has ever noticed me doing this to reassure you that something that feels so obvious to us can go completely under the radar for everyone else sharing the same space. But how can something so tiny make any difference?

*Draw a faint pencil line on a blank page, and you can hardly see it. Now keep making faint lines over and over, and watch as your page gradually changes in contrast. You can take it a step further if you like and keep the page on your workspace, drawing another single line each time you take a micropause. You may be surprised how quickly your pencil runs out of lead and requires sharpening.*

These three-second intervals, repeated often, literally become entrenched, helping you adopt a positive and relaxed mindset. They can be attached to almost anything you do. Simply pause, breathe in for three counts, gently let your breath go, and carry on. Each micro break momentarily returns you to the reality of each new moment as it unfolds. Repeating these micro pauses gently steers us away from our place behind the eight ball to where we can get a much clearer shot at our next challenge.

## BEFORE

*"Omg! It's awful! Everything is a struggle, and there is never enough time to get it all done. Even if I had an extra day, there would still be way too much to do. Why is it always me who has to do everything?"*

## AFTER

*"It's all pretty okay actually. Even if I do take on a lot, it doesn't all have to be done today. I can only do a day's work in a day. Anyway, I can always find someone else to help me. I don't have to do everything by myself."*

## WHAT WILL YOU PASS ON?

How would you like the home screen of your offspring to look? If there is anything about your own programming or the person you chose to have a child with that does not serve you well or aid your ability to function easily, you might want to rearrange it before you reproduce. If you already have children and notice some undesirable traits in yourself, it's still not too late to take responsibility for your actions and improve yourself moving forward. Everyone will benefit.

## WHAT DOESN'T CHALLENGE
## YOU WON'T CHANGE YOU

Parachutes and our minds work better once they are open. Whether it's putting the toilet seat down or the top back on the toothpaste tube, closing doors behind you, slowing down to the speed limit on the highway, responding rather than reacting, or pausing to listen instead of filling every conversational silence with your words, you will encounter some resistance when you begin changing. The bigger the pull to do something, especially if emotions are involved, the harder it will be to change. Any resistance is a good sign. When you are making these positive changes and receive negative backlash from someone else or from inside of yourself, see it as reassurance that what you are doing is working. This reprogramming can be as subtle as walking slightly slower, using a smaller plate to eat the same meal, using the three-second breath technique, or practicing the endless in breath, which I will explain later.

## FLAT-OUT OR FLAT OUT?

Do you feel driven to perpetually fill your personal calendar? Having this time-crippling program running all the time guarantees you will have no chance to rest. I call this flat-out or flat out because this perpetually busy lifestyle guarantees us to be either rushing around or lying in bed. This is usually driven by low self-esteem as we feel the need to explain to others why we can't do what they want us to do. We can also be terrified of looking bad by letting others down. By filling all of the gaps, we can wax lyrical about how full our day already is and how run off our feet we already are. Most of this seems to be done so that people will like us (which, of course, never works). And then there's the amplified gratitude from someone who knows how busy you were when you went out of your way to help them. A very effective way to counteract this debilitating programming is to make "me appointments."

## "ME" APPOINTMENTS

Once your me appointment is made, you can honestly say, "Sorry, I have an appointment already." No need to explain what it is about or who it is with. Once locked in, you can choose to cancel it if you wish, but you have the option. What you put in this new gap could be going for a walk or taking a short nap. If it's a walk you choose, then leave your device at home or in the car. The whole point of taking a gentle exercise break is to do a reset.

I take a thirty-minute nap every working day, which sets me up for a much more focused and present afternoon. NASA recently published the results of their study into daytime sleep. They discovered that the optimum length of time for a midday nap is twenty-six minutes.[3] If you are a red-liner, then your friends, workmates, family, and possibly your therapist may have suggested that you relax. But you soon realize that relaxing isn't something that can be "done."

## RELAXING CAN'T BE DONE

"Relax? No, I can't do that. I don't know how." Most requests made of us can be followed by an action. "Please pick the kids up from school today." "Kick the ball." "Pass the salt." "Would you mind going outside and grabbing a bunch of parsley from the garden?" These requests can all be followed by something that is done, but relaxing requires that we *don't* do something. Relaxation requires us to stop rather than do. Therefore, telling a person to relax is counterintuitive and confusing. What we can do is let go.

## LET GO

By letting go, we stop doing. During a treatment session, I ask my clients to first breathe in, activate certain muscle groups, and then let them go. In the half-hour treatment, this happens about twenty-five times. The act of letting go requires trust. As we let each breath go, we need to trust that we can take another. We release muscle tension in the knowledge that it can return at will. Each act of letting go, however subtle, drifts us closer to *having without holding*.

As a budding young entomologist, I was fascinated by insects as a child. I don't know if you have ever tried to hold onto a butterfly without doing it damage, but every time I caught one, I harmed it. No matter how careful I was, a leg would break off or some of its wing scales would rub off onto my fingers. But then I found one that had just emerged from its chrysalis. Having it stand unrestrained on my finger as its wings gained the strength to fly, I experienced freedom.

It's this way of being that most of the *human race* has lost. By making it a race, we have pressured ourselves. Applying the amount of

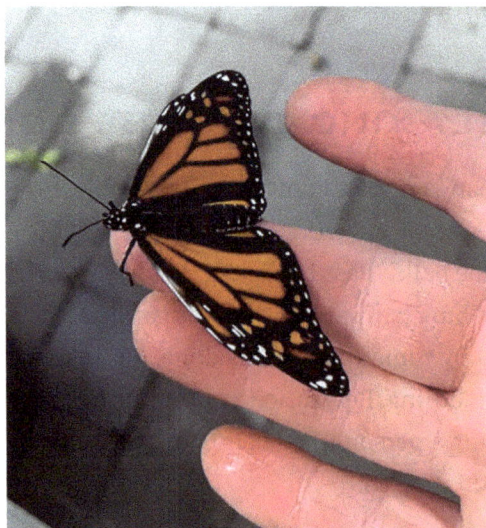

tension we currently see as normal or acceptable would squash the butterfly tightly inside our clenched fist, crushing it to death.

Indigenous cultures around the world once lived freely. A prime example is the aboriginal people, who for 60,000 years lived undisturbed. Traveling and living off the land, they made the first bread, were the first astronomers, and established the earliest records of religion. Their way of existence was systematically vacuumed up by the control, rules, regulations, beliefs, and pressures of the modern world. We introduced legal ownership and controlled systematic eradication of nature. We established exclusive systems requiring the pressure of enforcement. "I bought it and paid for it, so you all have to leave it alone and keep out!" Along with this ownership pressure came enforced belief in the form of exclusive organized religion. How does anyone promote an organization that has murdered tens of thousands of people in the name of its leader when the handbook clearly states, "Thou shalt not kill"? Talk about pressure and conflict! Most Western religions seem to be closed, exclusive franchises where there is the pressure of only one explanation of the "truth," which they own the rights to and are more than happy to sell to their followers. It was Martin Luther who, by translating the Latin bible into German, made it available to common people and pretty much single-handedly brought an end to the selling of forgiveness, which had become a popular revenue generator for the churches of the sixteenth century: "How relaxing would it feel, I wonder, to admit the actual 'truth,' which shall indeed 'set you free,' that no one knows any of this for sure. After all, why else would it be called faith?"[4]

It might reduce your own personal stress levels if you let go and enjoy yours without enforcing harm onto any more butterflies. I often wonder what is stopping us from treating each other well. Even if we could all manage to do nothing to anyone else that we would not have them do to us, the world would be transformed. But we don't.

The sad fact is that our society as a whole is moving steadily away from a peaceful, cooperative existence into hustle, bustle, noise, and greed. Like it or not, along with those things comes skyrocketing depression, anxiety, suicide, violence, physical disease, and associated pharmaceutical and recreational drug dependence. We are, as a society, becoming increasingly accustomed to the constant pressure of the red zone, with fight-or-flight engagement becoming a necessary and progressively acceptable part of everyday life. So, what happens in fight-or-flight mode anyway, and is it really all that bad for us?

# CHAPTER 9

# FIGHT-OR-FLIGHT

## COMMON LANGUAGE

*"I'm in a bit of a crisis."*
*"I feel a little bit terrified."*
*"My mind just went blank."*

## QUICK FIX

This intentionally fleeting survival mode system that is fight-or-flight, once engaged, alters all of your body's systems into elevated or reduced operations. It is useful on those rare occasions but harmful when left switched on. Take a breath, hold it in, then let it out slowly, or run cold water over your hands to disengage.

What is affected by our fight-or-flight response? The short answer is everything. A single drop of cortisol changes the blood chemistry, delivering an alert signal to every cell it comes into contact with. Your body's stress response triggers the release of sugars and increases blood pressure and heart rate, but there is a lot more to it.

Working as an advanced trade electrician for twenty years brought me into contact with some fascinating machinery, none less so than diesel-electric engine alternators. The company I worked for installed these in large buildings to keep essential communication equipment going during power failures. What does this have to do with the body and fight-or-flight mode? Even though these machines were huge, the installation and fuel cost of one large enough to run a whole building was prohibitive, so we split all of the building's wiring into two groups: essential and nonessential services. In the case of a power outage, one light was kept on in every room for staff safety; the rest of the available power supplied the technical equipment. All of the heating, most of the power outlets, and the rest of the lights were shut down.

Our bodies are wired in a similar way. In case of emergency, to maximize available energy reserves and optimize the performance of major muscle groups, all nonessential services are interrupted. Anything that is labeled as not necessary for survival in the next few minutes is either ramped down or turned off. The following is a list of warning signs from our bodies signaling fight-or-flight red-zone existence.

## DIGESTION

"Hmmm, a tiger on the loose and it's coming my way, think I'll finnish my sandwich before deciding what to do next. Hey mind with the claws, I'm still chewing!" It's just never going to happen like that is it. This situation would flick our fight or flight response totally on! The gut is designed to fire up again once any imminent danger has passed but when we are frightened, it shuts down. For anyone who leaves the alarm system a bit activated by something like an imminent deadline, digestion is compromised. Depending on how much stress we have learned to live with daily, the whole system could be running somewhere between reduced capacity and altogether off. The extreme is getting worried sick, which removes our stomach contents when we throw up. Unless food gets properly digested into tiny bits, it cannot get to where it is needed and therefore has zero opportunity to feed us. How small does it have to be? Microscopic. It's this system's partial failure that opens the door for the supplement industry. Because a large portion of our food is going in one end and out the other, we can become deficient. Some of what you then lack can be measured, and the rest is estimated, which means you can be administered daily dosages to replenish yourself. These you take in good faith, but they might not enter your bloodstream. If your digestive system is compromised by "a little stress," they, too, may pass right through.

## TASTE AND SMELL

These two senses are not required for immediate survival and therefore shut down. You won't be eating while your potential is to be eaten. If you find that your sense of taste or smell (or both) is diminishing, have a think about the amount of daily stress you have grown accustomed to. Any reduction in these senses can all too easily be written off as a natural part of the aging process. But you can probably fire these senses back up again simply by learning to live below the red line.

## VISION

To escape, you need to see where to go, so your long vision (distance) is really useful here. Your detailed, up-close vision is not as necessary in this panicked state. Even with poor close vision, you would still be able to see the shape of the tiger as it approached. You won't question a gradual reduction in your ability to see. Because it happens slowly to most of us in varying degrees, gradual vision impairment is also generally accepted as a normal part of the aging process. What we are gradually becoming more aware of is the fact that, yes, we are all getting older, and the aging process can cause deterioration, but we are at the same time being exposed to steadily increasing levels of daily stress. Long-term red-zone living can lock the eyes into malfunction.

## HEARING

Hearing serves no real purpose for fighting or running, so this gets added to the list of senses that are reduced while in fight-or-flight mode. It's mostly old people who wear hearing aids, right? This could easily be bundled into the same natural aging deterioration theory as the previous two examples. But not all old people need hearing assistance. It's more likely that those who do, have been living with their fear response set too closely to the red line.

## THE GUT RESPONSE

"It was horrific. I felt it in the pit of my stomach." Have you ever witnessed something that gave you a sudden lurch deep inside? These reactions are a signal that something is very wrong and digestion has been interrupted. There has been a lot of information circulating lately about the importance of gut bacteria: the wonderful, tiny gizmos that are essential to the health of our insides. Apparently, we need trillions of these microscopic digestion helpers, and altogether they can weigh more than our brain. The environment where they reside needs to be one in which they can flourish. But they can get totally wiped out. Garden plants require the correct balance of water, sunlight, nutrients, soil conditions, pest control, temperature, and location. Our internal flora is alive like a garden. Standing on thin ice, as the saying goes, inflames the gut environment, quickly wiping them out. There is a treatment available to boost the flora by taking some from a healthy gut and transferring them to the gut of a person who has low levels of healthy bacteria. This works really well in the short term because a thriving yet small community can be only established for a short time. But the environmental stress will kill them too.

### PETER

*"I've had so much trouble with my gut lately, having to eliminate an ever-expanding range of foods. That was until I went to the Islands for a two-week holiday. The longer I was there, the less it mattered what I ate.*

*Things that previously gave me a massive reaction were okay again. Two days after I got home and returned to work, my gut turned into custard again. I must be allergic to work!"*

## INFERTILITY

The stress of trying to get pregnant can make it less likely to happen. Maybe grandma was right when she said the best way to make a baby was to stop trying. David Attenborough often refers to the studies that have been undertaken on groups of animals where their environmental ups and downs are echoed in the number of births. When times are tough, the reproduction rates drop. Why would humans be any different?

A recent Endocrine Society Report states that overall, human fertility rates across the board have reduced by 50 percent over the last fifty years and is largely attributed to stress-reducing sperm counts, ovulation, and sexual activity. But science has found a way through. Through a number of avenues, the body's natural self-contraception stress response can be overridden, forcing conception. Considering evolutionary adaptations, will those children growing up in this negatively altered environment inherit a predisposition toward stress-related inflammatory diseases and infertility? Probably so.

## TAKING A NERVOUS ONE

Sheep and other prey animals, sensing danger, involuntarily empty their bladder. This lightens the load if running away, but urination also increases the chances of survival. Why? Because a full bladder under impact can burst, which would eventually result in an agonizing death. Maybe you've seen a movie where someone in mortal danger wets themselves? If you have been trotting off to do number ones a little more lately, maybe you have been fretting too much.

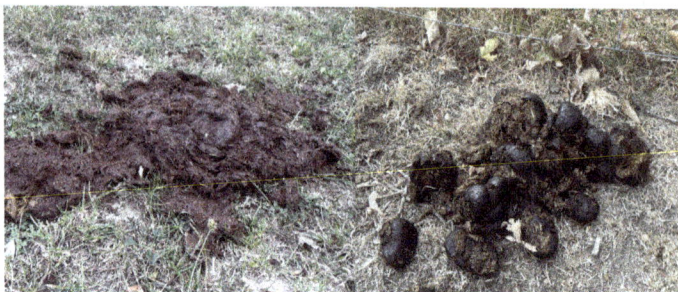

## GOT THE RUNS?

Ever heard people say, "It was a really scary situation. I was shitting myself the whole time"? Maybe you've heard, "Look at him! He's shit scared"? The reason diarrhea gets involved may come down to it being the quickest way to express solids (a further lightening of the load). I recently saw a young, relatively inexperienced horse after it was delivered to an unfamiliar property. After a one-hour ride alone in a horse trailer, the horse was understandably stressed and developed a bad case of diarrhea. Within two days, the horse's dropping went back to normal. So, if you've suddenly got the runs and you didn't eat some dodgy takeaway the night before, just remember the old saying, "This, too, will pass."

## MEMORY / CREATIVITY

In any panic situation, ruminating over what happened the last time a saber-tooth tiger peered into our cave, or planning different possible outcomes this time around, is useless. We just need to deal with the immediate threat or getaway. Stage performers know this memory shut-down only too well. Once the nerves kick in, the mind goes blank.

## SKIN

One of the other more obvious side effects is the reduction in skin color. Well-oxygenated blood is red, and when near the surface it is part of what gives the skin its healthy, warm glow. As the circulation is redirected to those areas most useful for survival, we can "look a little pale." Anything less than a healthy, warm glow could be an indicator that you are in the red zone.

## FEELING

Anyone who has ever had a serious accident will know that in the first few minutes after impact, there is very little pain or awareness of bodily damage. We definitely never need to know if we have been injured while fighting or running; therefore, pain reception is shut down. In the few minutes following any accident, the adrenaline leaves the bloodstream and we begin to receive pain signals again. "Oh yes. I thought I was all right, but now it feels like my leg might be broken." Much like the woman who was so stressed that she chopped the end off of her own finger while pruning roses. She had not felt the blade until it was too late. Living in a fight-or-flight mode as part of our daily reality not only dumbs us down but numbs us down as well and gives us the heightened tolerance to pain mentioned earlier.

## WORRIED SICK

This stress-related alteration of the body's systems makes it impossible to maintain homeostasis (a state of harmony and balance throughout the body). There are now billions of us all jammed in together, getting in each other's way. A visit to our local supermarket at their busy time has us competing at the carpark for a parking spot, dodging traffic on our walk inside, sharing each aisle with up to twenty others, and changing trolley directions up to ten times per aisle. The other constant disturbance is noise. I've recorded noise levels at a number of local cafes, and they average out at a staggering 80 decibels! (Hearing protection is suggested for anything above 85 decibels.) Roadside central city is in the high seventies. Alarmingly, even the supermarket records a steady low seventy decibels. This compares to being in nature, which is close to zero.

If accumulating societal stress and anxiety is causing you to suffer from any of the health complaints mentioned in this chapter, you may not have a short-term solution. Changes are usually difficult to make and typically harder to maintain, but it may help to know the possible causes. It is up to you what you will do next. One person cannot do everything to fix the current chaotic noise situation, but each of us can do something.

CHAPTER 10

# INFLAMMATORY DISEASE

## COMMON LANGUAGE

*"Don't do anything rash."*
*"A bit hot under the collar."*
*"Heated exchange."*

## QUICK FIX

Stifled emotional heat initiates internal dis-ease by highly sensitizing and inflaming tissues, which then hyper-react to low-level stimuli, reducing secondary infection resistance. Learn to safely express yourself. The truth withheld damages us internally. Once expressed it becomes a gift to the receiver and simultaneously one of self-healing.

We usually think of "dis-ease" (a state of being out of balance) as something that is capable of attacking the body from the *outside*. There are lots of viruses and pathogens that roam the globe, looking for a host—namely us! These diseases enter our bodies via water supplies, mosquitoes, contaminated food or water, animal-to-human contact, human-to-human contact, or even through the air we breathe. We accept that they all have the potential to invade our bodies and make us sick. But what about inflammatory diseases?

# "DIS-EASED"

If we were to pick and scratch at the wallpaper, looking for the hole that we know has to be there, this becomes a self-fulfilling prophecy when our picking wears through the surface and we actually make the hole. By worrying ourselves above the red line, we inflame ourselves. The further we are from being actively relaxed, the more we expose ourselves to the ill health of emotionally triggered inflammatory dis-eases. The most obvious of these has to be the skin. The integrity of our skin is essential to our survival. Apart from helping to contain our circulatory fluids, it also forms a very effective first defense barrier against invaders. Imagine working with your hands potting a plant or preparing a meal without your skin. Organs like the kidneys, liver, lungs, heart, and indeed every cell have a very thin skin or membrane covering and sealing them on their surface. The state of all of these skins can become compromised once we get a bit triggered.

Inflammation is useful in our bodies to aid healing by increasing the temperature to help kill unwanted viruses and bacteria. But this same response also weakens tissue. This is most obvious when it appears on our outsides with eruptions like psoriasis and eczema. These inflammatory outbreaks compromising our outer surface are easy to see. Our visible skin responds to any heightened emotional state by becoming warmer and reddened. The most obvious of these is blushing. When we are embarrassed, we get a bit flushed or red in the face. (Apparently there is now a surgical procedure available to disconnect the blush response.) Our necks tell a similar but usually much bigger story. When we have our *feathers ruffled*, some of us get a red neck. I have taken many photographs off reality television shows demonstrating this effect in action and chose two of the most dramatic to include as examples. Sadly neither of these photographs can be included for legal reasons so I will describe them instead. The first person had been triggered into a massive internal reaction, visible on the outside. Watching his conversational body responses with those around him gave very little indication that anything out of the ordinary was going on, but the color of his skin told an entirely different story. He had been triggered into a severe emotional response, suddenly turning the top of his chest and neck bright red. If you tune into any reality show, where the participants are involved in interpersonal conflict, you will be able to watch their exposed skin changing color. I'm not talking about sunburn here. Take a closer look at anyone involved in a *heated exchange* and you will notice their neck, arms and sometimes their entire upper body, turning red. The next subject is a young woman who began her interview with no sign of any skin discoloration on her almost completely exposed upper body. Within half a minute, while answering some very pointed and *potentially inflammatory questions*, her skin erupted in a grouping of large blotches. This blotching stood out clearly in a brightly reddened pattern like large spots on a leopard. Not confined to her neck, this emotionally charged skin response completely covered her shoulders, chest and arms as well. Again, just like the previous example, she gave no other obvious indication that she had been triggered. Sitting almost motionless with her arms folded, answering each question matter of factly as it arose.

This reddened glowing is skin inflammation that is evidence of "energy in motion," which is emotion made visible. Even though their skin color changes signal an intense reaction, they have each chosen to "keep a lid on things." If asked how they were feeling, they would more than likely use the most commonly told lie and answer, "I'm fine!" (The common definition of fine is Freaked-out, Insecure, Neurotic, and Exhausted.) Containerizing this surge of energy effectively turns the body into a *pressure cooker*. By choosing to "bottle up" our emotions inside ourselves, we are holding onto enormous amounts of heating energy on the inside. We choose how much, if any, of our true feelings make it to the surface, but the remainder is still in motion and needs to be containerized. Internalizing things that "make our blood

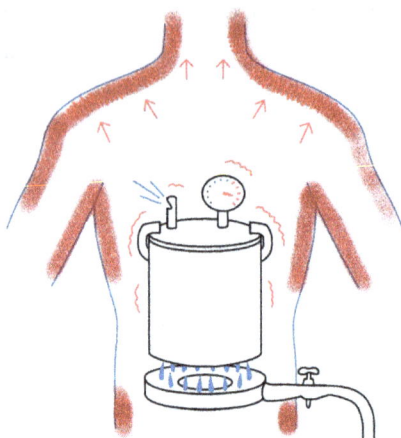

boil" or "give us a fire in our bellies" traps this energy where we can't see it.

The more time we spend outside of our comfort zones, the more heat is produced, adding to the container's pressure. In the case of burnout, the container is so pressurized for so long that it blows the lid off, distorting the surfaces and rupturing the seal. This is why it is crucial for us to "let off a little steam" or "vent our spleen." People with a jug boiling inside can waste an enormous amount of time and money searching for a cure for the ill health it causes. Our tissues, both internally and externally, echo all of the irritations and intolerances of the mind. Take a stroll around any chemist retailer and you will see row upon row of pharmaceuticals designed to help us cope with the fallout. The more we "see red" the hotter we get on the inside. You stand no more chance of having good health with your internal jug boiling than you do of picking up a boiling jug with your bare hands and not hurting yourself. This mechanism forms the basis of inflammatory diseases.

## INFLAMMATORY DISEASES

Louise Hay, the well-known pioneer of healing through mind-body recognition, listed the body locations affected by unresolved emotional energy in her book, *You Can Heal Your Life*. Food intolerances are usually the result of emotionally based intolerances. The digestive system is probably the most commonly inflamed internal area. The external redness visible on the neck also appears internally within the gut. These tissues cannot function normally while inflamed. A person who is open-minded and tolerant socially will have a lower flame than one who is reactive and more easily *aggravated*. Learning to be more *tolerant* and to accept the differences in others helps lower the flame under our pot, normalizing inflammatory responses, including the gut lining. Diverticulitis (an inflammation or infection in one or more of the digestive tracts) is not caused by an invasion of "diaverts." It is an *inflammatory dis-ease* of the digestive tract caused by a heightened emotional state. In other words, it is a "heated response." Once the lining of the gut wall inflames, it loses some of its integrity, and secondary irritations and infections are then a  given. This, along with irritable bowel syndrome,  are examples of internal reddening diseases and are initiated by long- term emotional upheaval.

The already aggravated gut lining in the drawing on the left has become highly reactive and intolerant. Foods that would pass through the gut on the right unnoticed would set off a chain reaction of responses

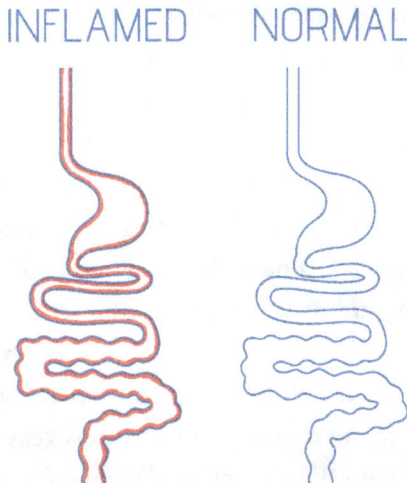

INFLAMED    NORMAL

in this preheated gastrointestinal tract. This is why we have to eliminate whole food groups from our diet just to keep from irritating this
emotionally inflamed tissue any further. It's not because we didn't like
the foods or that they were bad for us in any way; instead, our system,
with its already reddened tissue, was not able to handle any *further
irritation*. On our worst day, this has the potential to trigger a massive
reaction to very low stimulus commonly known as an *overreaction*.

## IMMUNE RESPONSE

If we worry obsessively, our mind is trying to fight off a threat that is
not present. This worry ignites our internal immune response, which
sends out our defense troops to search and destroy invaders. If these
troops, armed to the teeth, are continually dispatched to destroy an
invading force that is not actually there, they begin to destroy friendly
tissue. Interestingly, I have heard several similar accounts from clients with overactive immune response diseases where it has paused
for a week or two. Having suffered daily for decades, they were all
understandably amazed to have their symptoms disappear completely for the duration of their COVID-19 infections. Maybe the real
defense work given to the immune system was a big enough distrac-
tion for it to stop destroying the body. In all cases, the previously
debilitating symptoms returned once fully recovered from COVID-19.
As already mentioned in Chapter 9 on what we inherit, at least some
of these intolerances may not be caused by our own actions. Food
intolerances, just like other predispositions, may have been delivered
with the original IOS (internal operating system). Desensitizing yourself from these systems is possible. Elimination of food group reactions can be reprogrammed in a similar way in which someone can let
go of their fear of, say, spiders. By introducing incredibly small amounts
of a food that had previously brought about a reaction, the body's self-
defense radar learns not to generate a blip. Dosages can then be incrementally increased until the reaction is eliminated.

## THE PRESSURE GAUGE

There is a pressure gauge on the back of your neck. I have included a series of images of these. This reddening gives a visual moment in time, indicative of your internalized pressure.

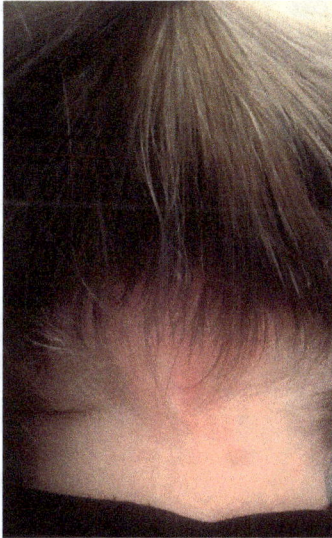

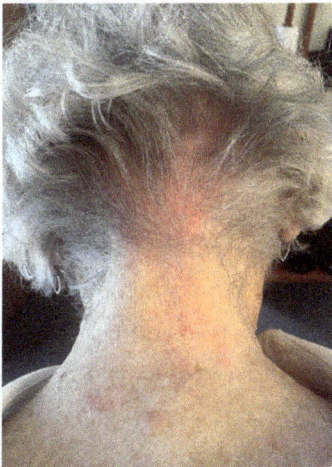

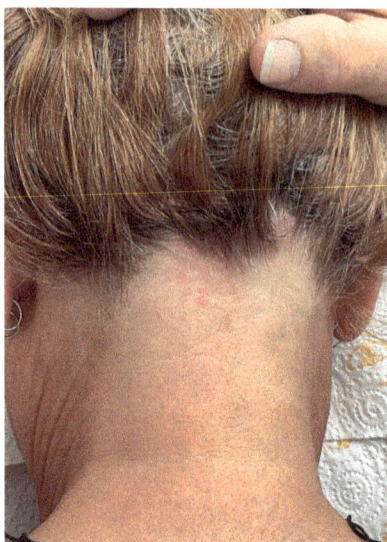

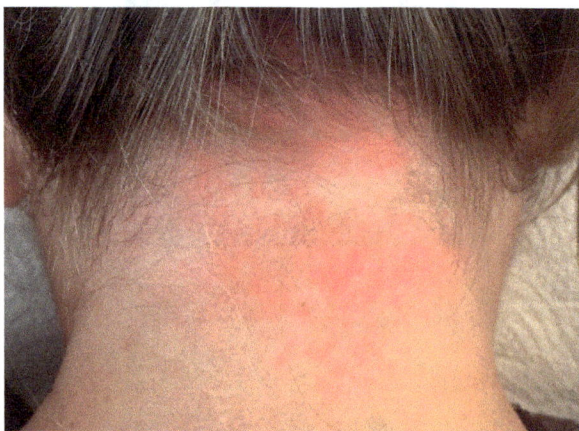

Red necks and chests are more transitional, but these in the photos are semi-permanent. You will have seen these irritation indicators in action on the screen when an actor raises their hand to gently scratch the skin on the back of their neck with their fingers. They do this to convey a feeling of *irritation* by another. Maybe you have felt this in yourself during *prickly conversations* in reaction to a person saying something annoying. They are always in the same spot in the center, right at the top of the neck. A large part of the work I have done over the years has been focused on necks and shoulders, mainly because this is one of the body's favorite places to hold a bit of tension. Turns out that the people who needed me most often had this same indicator. From little rows of what looked like pimples to large, reddened blotches, you could say a pattern was emerging. Of even more interest were the few indicators that changed. It turned out that the more stressed each person had become, the more the back of their neck got inflamed. One person in particular had a fairly calm-looking area of slight discoloration that would occasionally morph into an eruption closely resembling psoriasis, every time coinciding with a particularly stressful event. At each of these events, the reddened area also expanded out from a golf ball diameter to that of a softball. These blotches, each with their own individual shapes, color, and sizes, indicate an excess of internalized heat energy.

## INTERNALIZED HEAT ENERGY

By swallowing down your feelings, you are trapping energy inside in the form of heat. This heat generates all of the same skin breakouts internally as those that are visible on the outside. Conditions like eczema, rashes, and psoriasis (once internalized) appear on organs and hidden skins. Everything inside you is wrapped in a type of skin, and it is these tissues that are compromised in the presence of sustained emotionally generated inflammation. We all run the risk of developing any one of a long list of inflammatory diseases, where the causes are currently listed as unknown. If an internal site started to break down as a consequence of this prolonged emotionally based inflammation, then as long as the stimulant was present the symptom would be sustained or further deteriorate. Any one of these inflamed internal surfaces or skins could be the next one to erupt, and lose it's integrity. Once this protective seal becomes compromised, it leaves any affected area open to the possibility of secondary infection. The worst of these internal disturbances has the potential to transition into cancer.

# MENINGITIS

Meningitis is an infection of the fluid and membrane around the brain and spinal cord. This potentially life-threatening disease can get a foothold because of the stress-related inflammation of the surrounding tissues. Meninges are the tri-layered protective skins covering these most sensitive of our organs. Their job is to contain, seal, and protect the contents. To do this, meninges need to have structural integrity. As exposure to things that we call a "pain in the neck" build, inflamed neck tension develops. This localized inflammatory response is then transferred to the spinal cord tissue, degrading the surface sufficiently to invite infection.

# EAR INFECTIONS

There is a rather long group of muscles rising out of the base of the spine at the center of our pelvis, traveling all the way up to eventually attach right next to our ears. I call them the horse's reins because we are meant to slow down when we feel them pull. The trouble for our ears begins when we, like some horses, "grab the bit between our teeth" and keep going. Tapping into the earlier analogy of our internal pressure cooker, steam gathers right beside our ears, overheating the ear canals, which, just like the spinal cord, lose their integrity and become infected. This ongoing irritation also triggers the release of extra ear wax which is the body's way of attempting to resolve the issue.

Animals also have the horse's rein muscles. They, too, suffer from stress-related ear infections. Cats, dogs, and horses can have their symptoms eased or even eliminated with a bit of gentle hands-on treatment. You can ease their suffering by massaging and stretching their necks. The offending muscles are relatively easy to locate,

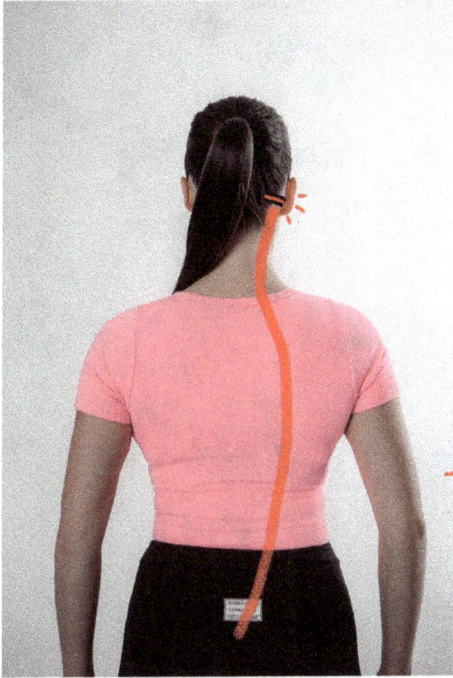

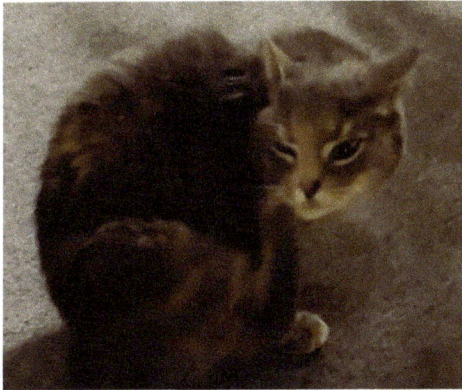

running from behind their ears to the tops of their shoulders. The solution to all emotionally fueled inflammatory diseases is the same: Breathe fully and slowly, calming the body by calming the mind. This next chapter takes a close look at why it is such a challenge for us to fully integrate this seemingly simple health-enhancing technique.

# CHAPTER 11

# BREATH OR DEATH

## COMMON LANGUAGE

*"It was like someone had sucked the air out of the room."*
*"I'm just holding my breath until I know*
*for sure what's going to happen."*
*"It was like a breath of fresh air."*

## QUICK FIX

Improve your general health by up to 75 percent with diaphragmatic "tummy balloons." This disengages the flight-or-fight response, returning your body systems to normal operation. This fully functional relaxed breathing optimizes gas exchange, detoxifying abdominal organs while returning your body systems to normal operating levels.

As a teenager, I pondered how two pieces of toast and Marmite were enough to keep my body going throughout a morning of physical activity. Much later in life it dawned on me: I was breathing in fuel in the form of oxygenated air the whole time! When our full respiratory system is underutilized or not in top working order, we are robbing ourselves of vital fuel. With diminished respiratory function everything, even the smallest task, becomes an effort. We are collectively spending a fortune on health-enhancing food supplements, but how much would you pay for a single thing that could improve your health across the board by a staggering 75 percent? You can forget the rest. Fully functional diaphragmatic breathing can improve your overall health by up to 75 percent all at once. Plus, it's free! How did I decide it was 75 percent? It's purely mechanical. This is the portion of our breathing potentially done by our breath-exclusive muscle group, the diaphragm.

For a system that is automatically regulated, controlled breathing, whether conscious or subconscious, is more often than not at the center of bodily dysfunction. It's important for us to have an internally regulated system of breathing because it is essential to our survival. If left entirely to us, we could simply forget to breathe and of course, death would quickly follow. We can live for up to three months without food but only minutes without taking a breath.

Our respiration follows our feelings, reflecting happiness, sadness, frustration, anger, joy, and grief. Any situation that generates a negative emotion has a tendency to initiate holding, stifling, or fixation in our breathing patterns. The more joy-filled moments trend more toward opening, softening, and relaxation. If you want to keep the air in a balloon that is not tied, you have to squeeze the neck firmly shut. And so it is with holding our breath. This holding has to happen in the surrounding structures of the throat diaphragm or rib cage because all of the parts that make up the breathing tubes and lungs are passive. Not all holdings are the same. We, depending entirely on the type of emotional trigger, can hold our breath either in or out.

*To construct a visual example of a passive lung, wrap a kitchen sponge in plastic cling wrap and pop a hole in one side by inserting a drinking straw. When you squeeze the sponge, air will exit through the tube. Release the pressure, and the air is drawn back in.*

The lungs, absent of contractile tissue, are incapable of breathing by themselves. They wait to be inflated or deflated in response to the movement of the surrounding structures. If you installed the sponge and

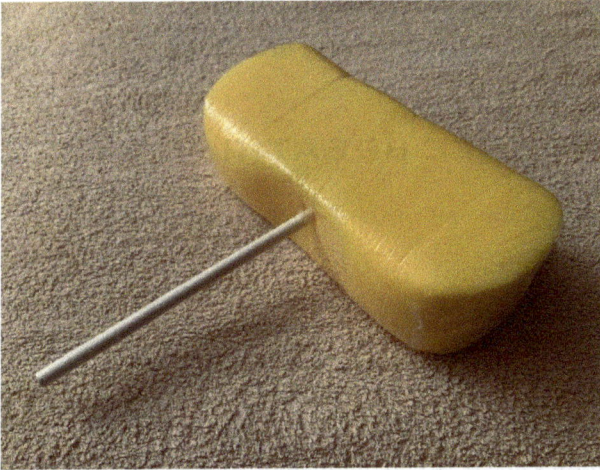

drinking straw into a musical squeeze box and sealed it tight except for the straw, the sponge would draw in and express air as the two ends are pulled apart and squeezed back together. This is how our lungs work. The tube connecting the lungs up to our mouth is flexible but rigid, like the drain hose on washing machines. It is not possible to restrict air flow anywhere along this tubing but there is a controllable flap at the back of our throat. This is where some of us create back pressure.

*Breath in and out as quickly as you can through your mouth. The amount of sound generated reflects the extent of your throat's holding. To locate these air-constricting muscles, repeat the breathing, only this time as noisily as you can. Then, relaxing the muscles you have just found, repeat the breaths with the same intensity as quietly as you can.*

Next time you tune in to watch the news or weather report on the TV, have a listen for tight-throated breathing sounds. Some presenters can be very clearly heard rasping their in-breath. The reporters who do this will also be holding the microphone with white knuckles and gasping teaspoon-size breaths midsentence. This stress induced sentence chopping they do to gasp in some air is now a trend, which I am guessing will soon be common enough to be accepted as normal phrasing.

Unfortunately for us, we are free to select healthy or unhealthy breathing patterns because we have three breathing systems to choose from.

## THE THREE BREATHING SYSTEMS

The first and the worst of these three systems pull the tops of your lungs a tiny bit upward. If you have ever watched an asthmatic using their inhaler, you will have seen this system in action. The second breathing system expands the ribcage a little sideways. The third system, vastly superior and highly efficient, draws a massive breath down.

I've decided to bunch the first two together because of how similarly inefficient they are. Between them, these inferior systems utilize approximately ninety-six joints and sixty muscles to inflate the lungs to a miserable 25 percent of their full capacity. All of this they achieve by moving the ribs. If you are already proficient with utilizing system three, then this next exercise does not apply to you but most of us are not!

*Stand in front of your bathroom mirror and take in a huge breath. There isn't much to see at first because the air is mostly being drawn sideways. Keep going, and near the end of this breath you will see your shoulders rise, your chest lift, and the muscles on the front and sides of your neck standing out.*

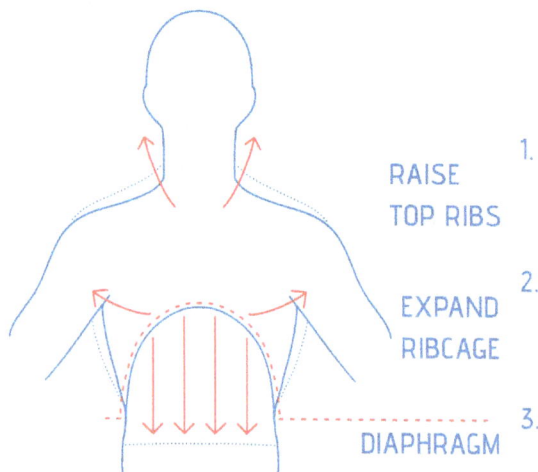

1. RAISE TOP RIBS

2. EXPAND RIBCAGE

3. DIAPHRAGM

If you are keen enough to look it up you can see a great example of neck muscles lifting the top ribs in the movie *Queen of the Desert*.[1] Halfway through the movie, Nicole Kidman acts out a scene involving intense grief in which her neck muscles are literally a stand out!

*To feel the second of these two systems operating, place your hands flat on either side of your ribcage as you take in another big breath. You may feel all of your ribs expanding out and a little upward.*

There is a pretty good chance you will not feel anything unfamiliar because even though it is hopelessly inefficient, most of us now breathe this way. So, what is driving us to breathe up and sideways? As our society becomes progressively fear-based and collectively unaware of our third breathing apparatus, we only *think* we have a need for more air. It all began some 200,000 years ago when our ancestors got scared. All they had for shelter and protection would have been a hole in the side of a cliff without a door. Exposed to attack from huge predators, they found a way of maximizing their strength by increasing their breathing capacity. They did this by recruiting minor muscle groups that expanded and lifted their rib cage. After nearly two hundred thousand years of living this way, this stressed breathing adaptation became deeply embedded into our subconscious minds. Present-day living, with the saber-tooth tigers long gone, we have overlaid this prehistoric default setting into our collective fear of everyday life. Struggling to get enough air in and unaware of our third breathing system, we alarmingly *run out of options*.

## RUN OUT OF OPTIONS

What was originally developed as an add-on to increase lung capacity has become our default setting. Fear-response breathing used to be just that. Each external attack would have triggered a collective stress response, but only while the threat was actually present. As long as the fire was blazing in the cave entrance and the whole family was safely inside, everyone would have breathed easily. As we incorporate more red-line living into daily life and hold onto our unexpressed feelings deep down inside, we lose the relaxed breathing style altogether. Now we rely exclusively on what used to be an *emergency-only system*. What this means for us is the shocking reality that our threat, imagined or not, is now constantly present! I have already mentioned that breathing up and out by moving our ribs is hopelessly inefficient, but this situation gets worse the more we rely on it. The muscles we recruit to breathe in this way were designed to move our head and neck around and enhance mobility by moving our ribs apart and together like a concertina. Because of this occasional use, their tissue is like the other body movement muscles, which are prone to fatigue. The third system's muscle tissue is more like that of our heart, which is designed to work repeatedly throughout our life. We take somewhere near twenty-two thousand breaths every day, which is why this breathing muscle group has to be different. You are not capable of turning your head that many times in one day because your neck muscles would fatigue and seize up. But we expect these same muscles to keep raising our ribs all day every day. Under repetitive use and laboring, the neck and rib muscles increasingly hold tension and tend to compact and lock short. This locks the ribs at the top of their swing. Without breath we die, and the added stress of struggling to breathe into a system that is failing, creates its own tension, which makes breathing even more difficult. For most of us, this shortness of breath becomes little more than a constant inconvenience as we struggle to function normally with reduced cardiovascular performance. At the top end of this scale are panic attacks and asthma.

## MARY

*"It feels amazing. Now that you've got my breathing freed up, I can do my turns in the pool now without feeling panicky."* Restoring the movement into what Mary called her "tin-can chest" took her breath capacity from close to zero up to somewhere nearer 25 percent. This improvement, although comparatively subtle, felt dramatic, and she was thrilled to be "breathing normally again." Mary still had no idea that

she had probably never used the other 75 percent.

This sounds dire, but an alarming number of people have been chronically breath restricted for so long that they have no idea that something like two and a half of their three options for staying on the planet have almost totally failed! Hypoxia, a condition resulting from reduced blood oxygen levels, has been tested on deep-sea divers in controlled pressure tanks. Testing each individual's ability to operate while exposed to a reduction in available oxygen, the results showed an interference with normal brain function. Extreme testing revealed that those people who had their oxygen levels reduced sufficiently lost the ability to perform even the most basic of tasks. This helps to explain why other apparently unrelated health issues disappear once breath is restored. You've waited long enough, so let's delve into the magic of . . . system three.

## SYSTEM THREE

Everyone is certainly familiar with their bicep muscles. Reading the word *bicep* has probably already created an image in your mind of a bulging muscle that sits between the elbow and shoulder.

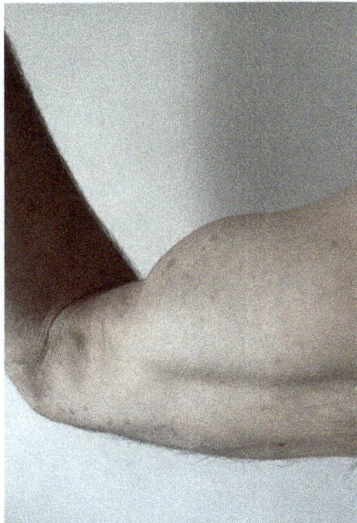

More often than not, the mental image that appears in response to reading the word *diaphragm* looks more like a large blank space with a question mark in the middle.

## INTRODUCING, THE DIAPHRAGM

Courtesy of a local home-kill butcher, the diaphragm pictured here is from a sheep's carcass. The camera angle is upward from the base of the ribs toward the neck. One side of the lung is clearly visible through the non-muscular window section. You will have to imagine the other half as this image shows only one of two equal parts. Because you can never see your diaphragm, tucked away inside the base of your ribcage, it is difficult to fully understand. Even though its name is singular, it is made up of twelve individual muscles, all working together. There is a tidal wave of information surfacing at the moment

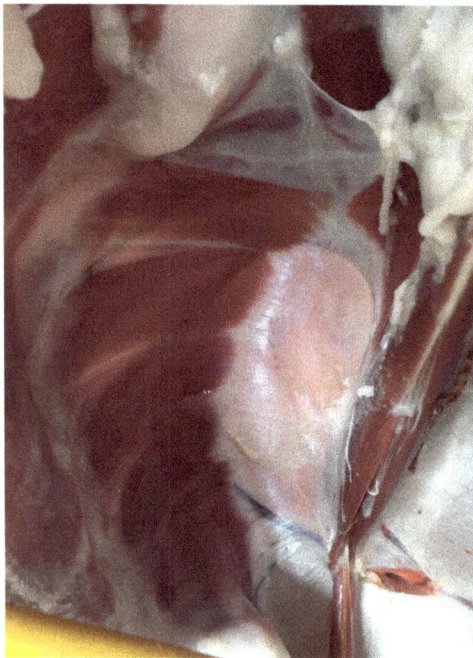

about the incredible health benefits of breathing through your nose instead of your mouth. This latest health trend is sure to become a global phenomenon. Backed by screeds of testing and long lists of proven results, this amazing rediscovery almost misses the most important fact. Nose breathing switches off breaths one and two and engages your diaphragm. So then, where is our diaphragm, and how does it work? To get a visual impression, I like to use pudding bowls and dinner plates.

*Trace the outer attachments of your diaphragm by running your fingertips around the bottom edge of your ribcage. This outer edge rigidly holds the shape while creating the seal. Now imagine a pair of upside-down pudding bowls, side by side inside your ribcage, joined across the middle with their bottom edges along this perimeter. This is how your diaphragm looks in the off position. Switch it on and it pulls down flat and looks like a pair of dinner plates. Our lungs inflate and deflate by following these up and downward movements, producing the other 75 percent of our full lung capacity.*

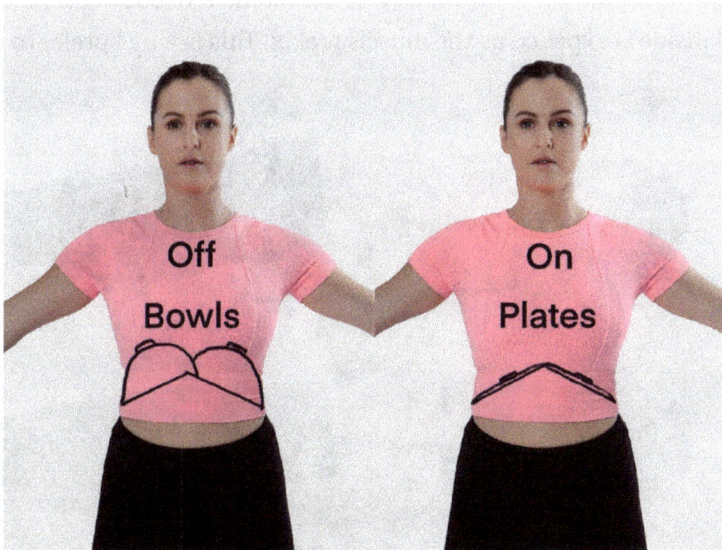

*You can't fail this next test. If your diaphragm is working properly, you just need to keep your mouth shut to keep engaging it; if not, you have huge potential for better overall health. Place one hand on your chest and the other on your belly while taking a few full breaths. The hand that moves has found the direction of your breathing. If you find your tummy hand moving very little or not at all, you have been red-lining your body into a state of unrest. You can reinvigorate your diaphragm and calm your whole self by doing tummy balloons.*

## TUMMY BALLOONS

*Lie on your back, placing both of your hands gently on your tummy. With eyes closed and lips held gently together, breathe in through your nose, feeling your tummy rising. It may be a little easier at first to imagine the air is entering your body through your belly button. Release all of the air but only when it stops going in.*

I used the word *release* here because using the diaphragm to breathe only requires the muscles to switch on and off again. *There is never any need to force the air out.* At the moment of our death, the air held inside is expelled as the muscles relax. This is why I prefer to call

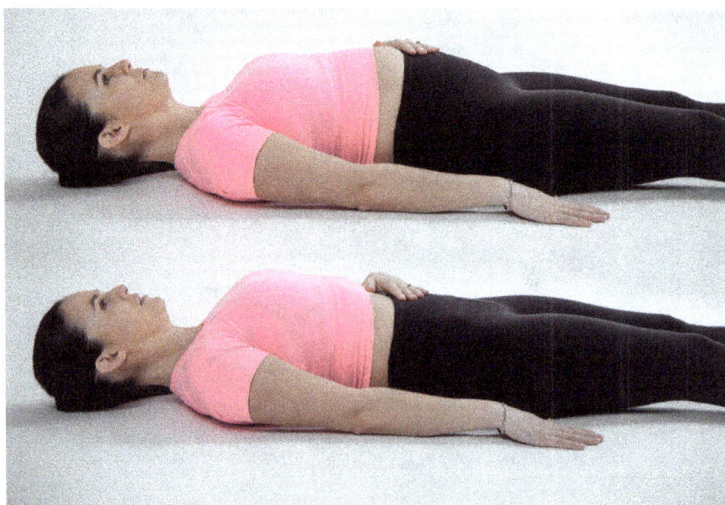

it *breathing in and letting go*, because the only effort ever required is to get the air in, and of course letting go is something we could all benefit from a little more of.

If you want to be a fit strong athlete, you have to do a training program designed to incrementally increase your performance. These same principles apply here. To transform your diaphragm muscles from the thickness of a paper towel to about as thick as your little finger, you need to do a regular workout. A gentle word of warning first: If you haven't done much exercise and you suddenly go for a ten-kilometer walk (around six miles), two days later your legs will be so painful it'll be hard for you to move. The same principle applies to your diaphragm. It too is a muscle group, so while rehabbing, a little exercise each day is the best way to avoid the pain of rehabilitation gain. A good start is to do ten slow full-tummy balloon breaths twice daily. This will help you to avoid the stitch.

## THE STITCH

Although shrouded in mystery, the stitch is nothing more than a cramp in one of the diaphragm's muscle bellies. It's an easy fix. *Take in as much air as you possibly can and go into a squat (see image overleaf). Hold this position as long as you comfortably can. You will find it a lot easier to do if you hold onto something like a post and pull back slightly as you crouch. This way, you will be able to drop a little lower. Breathing in activates the muscles, and the squeeze from the abdominal contents gives them a gentle stretch, releasing the muscle spasms.*

## THOSE ROCK-HARD ABS HAVE TO GO

Abs look sexy, and it's cool to have them flexed, but not all of the time. In order for this big double piston to travel down toward the pelvis, it needs somewhere to go; whatever was previously occupying the space

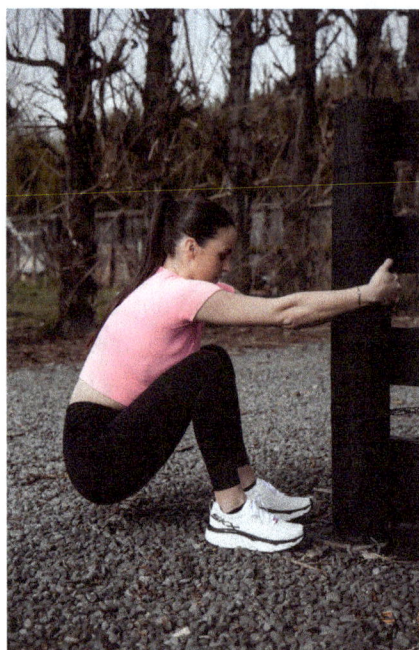

has to move out. The pelvis and spine are solid structures and cannot move out of the way, so that rules out movement down and back. The only option left for the abdominal contents is to go forward. As you have already discovered, your tummy has to expand to accommodate the movement. It has to be soft to do this. If you walk around holding your tummy flat so you can look good, *then you shut the whole process down.*

*Once you have your tummy balloons working well, poke your finger into your soft tummy, then switch your abs on so that they push your finger out. Now, holding your finger there to make sure the abs stay locked on, try and take a deep diaphragmatic breath.*

Mary was working overseas as a professional dancer, and it had become exhausting. She said she always felt short of air. She explained she had been taught to always hold her tummy tight. This, the teachers explained, was not only to display perfect posture; it gave the male dancers a firm surface with which to hold them. A lot of the time she thought she was going to pass out during a show or rehearsal. This ridiculous situation sets dancers up to fail and must surely be the only intense physical activity that is begun by intentionally restricting breathing capacity! An even worse scenario is to attempt ballroom dancing while wearing a corset. Not only do these laced-up body prisons shut the diaphragm down completely; they also stop the ribs from expanding outward. It's little wonder their breasts would heave upward at the slightest provocation; the poor souls were trying to stay alive. With the belly and ribs tightly bound, it was left to the neck muscles to drag in teaspoons of air by forcing the top three or so ribs to lift.

## RESTORATION

There are a few instances where the spinal bones at the rear of the ribcage have been strangled for so long that they have begun to break down, but for most of us, the potential to breathe fully is still intact. In the case of the "tin can" mentioned earlier, the ribs had all jammed in the up position, incarcerating the upper spine. This not only restricts breath but movement as well.

My client Mary Fox Turnbull, associate professor at the University of Waikato in New Zealand, sent me this feedback. *"I first went to Alistair three months ago with very sharp pains in my neck and shoulder area. After a month of intensive treatment, I noticed several improvements, which have continued since. I have sports- induced asthma and often take my peak flow measurement. This has improved by approximately 75 to 100 points since beginning treatment with Alistair."*

## MARY

Initial assessment revealed Mary's jammed mid to lower ribcage and upper spine, with severely compacted muscles throughout her neck. Together, these dysfunctions were almost completely shutting down her ability to utilize the two minor breathing systems she had learned to rely on. Also, the anterior neck muscle compactions were support-

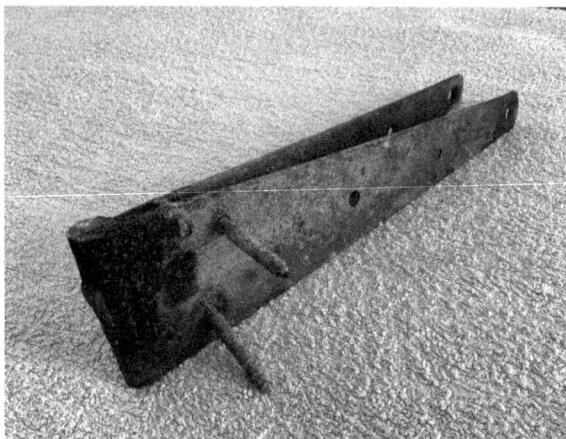

ing pressure point activity, radiating painful referrals to her shoulders. The treatments restored full, natural movement to all of the joints and full range of motion to her neck muscles. In doing so, the pressure points and subsequent shoulder pain referrals were eliminated. All that was left to do was introduce Mary to her diaphragm.

This rusty gate hinge could be restored to near-perfect operation with a little TLC. When Mary first presented, her thoracic skeleton was stuck, just like this hinge. If you gave the gate attached to this hinge a kick to get it open, either the hinge would snap or the screws would pull out. But a wee wiggle and a bit of CRC lubricant and it would begin to move. Keep gently wiggling and lubricating and the gate would eventually swing freely. Treatments combined with some very simple breathing homework provided Mary's wee wiggle, and of course the CRC was her blood supply, which flooded back in the moment movement was reinitiated. Mary's breathing homework was to do multiple daily endless in breaths and tummy balloons.

## ENDLESS IN BREATHS

This breathing restoration technique is easy, free, and can be done anywhere at any time. All you do is breathe in without stopping. By continuing to breathe in, everything goes a fraction further than it was before, initiating a tiny bit of movement into all of your frozen respiratory joints and muscles. Don't be too surprised if you get a little sore around the ribcage in the early stages of your breath recovery. This will, like your diaphragm, be the muscles between all of your ribs and along your spine waking up after years of inactivity. The more you do this exercise the easier it gets, like blowing up a new balloon.

In a similar way to the previous diaphragm restoration technique, all you focus on is gently breathing in through the nose with the mouth closed. The difference this time is you don't stop. Keep breathing in, even though it feels like nothing is happening. Keep going for as long as you possibly can and then release. If you begin to feel panicky, huff a few quick noisy out breaths to reset. Do not at any stage hold your breath in by closing the back of your throat. As you use this method to progressively reawaken the dormant areas of your full breathing capacity you will, if you keep going, eventually discover the miracle that is total-body breathing.

## TOTAL-BODY BREATHING

You will probably find this technique quite difficult the first few times you try, but as your endless in-breathing draws air deeper into your respiratory system, it is sure to wake up every sleeping corner of your dormant lung capacity. It will be hard to find the muscles and difficult to breathe into that unfamiliar space. Persevere and you will eventually feel the effect spread out to include your whole body. Each full in-breath slightly increases your internal body fluid pressure, which drops down again as you exhale. It may help to imagine this as the rising and falling of the ocean's tides or waves on the beach. The pressure drop of each complete out-breath assists the body fluid's return to your heart. You will get signals from your body to let you know that what you are doing is working. At about the one-minute mark, there will be a tingling feeling that starts around the back of your neck. You can, by increasing the intensity a little, spread this reawakening to the top of your head, out into your fingers, and down to your toes. This sensation signals increasing vitality as you become more alive. There is a significant side benefit to all of your newly found breathing capacity, which may surprise you. It's what I call a breath-powered organ detox.

## BREATH-POWERED ORGAN DETOX

Positioned directly below the diaphragm are the liver, kidneys, stomach, and spleen. A little farther down are the large intestine and pancreas. These top four are not just near the underside; they are right up against it. As the breath is drawn in and the lungs expand downward, that soft area commonly known as the stomach is pushed forward. This is more than obvious, especially if the in-breath is taken quickly. What happens, under our radar, is all of these organs becoming gently squeezed and released with each fully functional breath. The diaphragmatic in-breath can be deep enough to completely displace all but the kidneys down to a new position and, when released again, allow them to travel right back up to where they were.

*By only breathing up, we rob these organs of this essential detoxifying massage!*

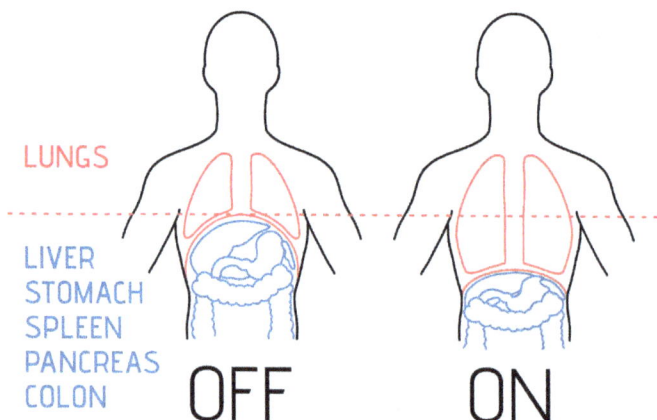

LUNGS

LIVER
STOMACH
SPLEEN
PANCREAS
COLON          OFF                    ON

Try to clean a dirty sponge or cloth under the tap without giving it a few squeezes, and most of the rubbish stays inside. We squeeze the sponge to clean it, which is exactly what happens to our organs when the diaphragm compresses and releases them from above.

## REFLUX & BLOOD PRESSURE

Seeing how the diaphragm squeezes the stomach makes it easy to understand why you should never leave your diaphragm switched on. I mentioned earlier that we control our emotions by holding breath either in or out. If you are *"just holding it all together,"* you may very well be causing reflux by squeezing your stomach contents back up your esophagus. You may also be holding enough breath tension to strangle the rest of your upper organs. Your spleen holds your spare blood, so squeezing it raises your blood pressure, but this compression also hampers circulation. This blood-filled balloon works alongside your heart. Every complete outwards breath reduces internal pressure in your spleen which assists the blood's return from your extremities. You will have cold feet and hands if your spleen is perpetually compressed from above. Another sign of your breath being held tightly in, may be spotting of the facial skin and around the base of the neck as your liver signals its compressed distress.

## CONTROLLING PANIC

Most people would rather swim with sharks than speak in public, so I guess that makes it one of our biggest fears. Mary originally came to me with excruciating mid- to lower back pain, which would be best described as extreme. The intensity of this pain had her calling out and freezing whenever she attempted to sit up from a lying down position. With an overall spinal mobility of about 25 percent, it was not surprising that her back had finally "gone out" while bending forward into a small vehicle. After a number of weekly sessions, her spine returned to a more functional 75 percent of full mobility, and her back pain was completely gone. Feeling much improved, with the back pain resolved, it was then that Mary said that she would give anything for her dizzy spells to be gone. I know from experience that compaction and joint stiffness in the upper neck can cause dizziness, particularly in cases where concussion has been diagnosed (more on that later). So, in search of a solution, I went about releasing the accumulated neck and shoulder tension. With this restoration almost complete and no obvious improvement, Mary told me that she had felt very dizzy twice in the past two weeks, and both times she had been in public situations involving interaction with large groups of people. She also said that as well as feeling dizzy she had temporarily lost some of her memory, had vision reduction, and experienced a "hurricane" in her head along with a "spiky" brain fog.

This revelation warranted an investigation into her breathing patterns. I videoed her lying on her back while taking three big breaths. All of her breath was going up! This was fantastic news because it meant her potential to improve as far as her diaphragm was concerned was 100 percent. I explained to Mary that the more we panic, for whatever reason, the more the breath forces upward until the top ribs jam against the collar and neck bones. This accelerates the panic, further opening the fight-or-flight tap. The beginning of Mary's solution was to assist her to first find and then reinvigorate her diaphragm. Once located, she agreed to a twice-daily rehab program of twenty gentle breaths through the nose.

There is a huge variation in the intensity of panic attacks, the worst of which present with drenched full-body sweating, racing heart, shortness of breath, memory loss, visible shaking, paralysis, and even possible fainting. What Mary was experiencing sounded about halfway up the scale. Mary could now avoid these attacks

intensifying or even diffuse their symptoms by using her newly rees-
tablished diaphragmatic breathing. The next stage was to get Mary
endless in-breathing into her "tin can" to free it all up. She returned to
her next session overjoyed. Having done her breathing exercises dili-
gently, reinvigorating her diaphragm, she had already been successfully using it to ease her symptoms. Once reinvigorated, you can
utilize your own diaphragmatic breathing to tune into your seventh
sense: breathing.

## SEVENTH-SENSE BREATHING

Most of us already know about our five senses. Less well recognized
is our sixth sense which tells us where our body is and, more impor-
tantly, where our limbs are.

*Stand up with your eyes closed and move one of your arms up,
down, forward, and back. There is no trick to this; you can tell where
your arm is all the time. What you are using is your positional
sense. Most of us have been unaware of this sense even though we
use it every day.*

Our seventh sense is also positional and another we are probably
unaware of. The difference is, this one tells us where we are centered
in relation to our physical self between our head and the center of our
body. Imagine a ladder inside of you, from the top of your head all the
way down to the center of your abdomen. This seventh sense tells you
which ladder rung you are on. You can learn to ascend or descend by
sitting still and focusing on your breath. I like to stay away from suggesting that anyone meditate because so much meaning has been
attached to this word. It can easily turn into a kind of spiritual Olym-
pics where the goal is to have dramatic experiences away from the
physical body by traveling off to realms far away and meeting up with

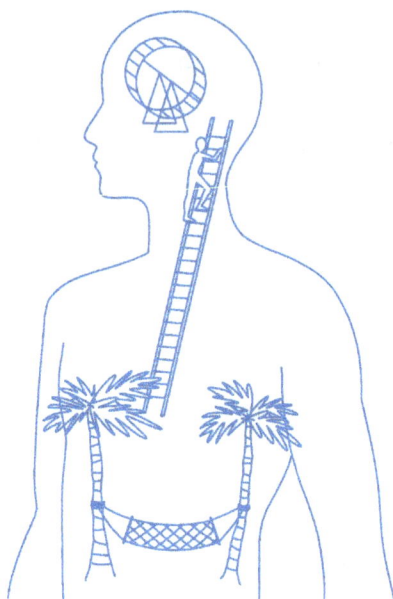

ethereal beings in our different head space that will tell us what to do next. Our stress-related diseases are already initiated by us distancing ourselves from our bodies as we *"jump out of our own skins"* or become *"beside ourselves."* Living in your head by adventuring even farther from your body center is like becoming a passenger in your own car. The place to be is at the base of your ladder in the driver's seat where you can operate your own vehicle. Your body will never tell you a lie and always knows what you need to do next. All you ever need to do is listen.

> *Sit comfortably with your mouth gently closed and focus on your breathing.*

That's it! You will begin to notice where you are on your ladder and learn to breathe yourself closer to your *home* state (or balanced state). There is really no more to it. I know we all want it to be a lot more complex. We are conditioned to buy gadgets, eat special foods, and buy the latest paraphernalia to improve our health. But there is not a single thing better for your overall health than incorporating this seventh-sense awareness breath technique into your everyday life.

Chapter 12 looks into how we allow the unrelenting pressures of our modern society to change us, why it causes our breathing to become and stay dysfunctional, and how this negatively impacts our body.

# PRESSURE: THE UNDERLYING CAUSE

## COMMON LANGUAGE

*"I've bitten off more than I can chew."*
*"I'm relaxed on the outside, but on the inside I'm a mess."*
*"Just barely holding it all together."*

## QUICK FIX

Becoming reasonably comfortable with continued exposure to dangerously unhealthy levels of life pressure negatively impacts all body systems. Compaction, allowed to silently accumulate, spreads through the body like a wildfire of pain, generating internal destruction. Fire up your tummy balloons as your first line of defense.

Humans are the only animals who choose to override their natural instincts. "Putting on a brave face" and operating under a "manageable level of stress" is now an acceptable part of mainstream society. For an increasing number of us, this goes on all day, every day, and even while we toss and turn at night. Having progressed away from the village way of life, we go it alone. With village living, the support network is a given. All of the people work and play for the common good, making sure everyone gets less of what they want and more of what they need. This is a constant from newborn babies right through to the end of life. Childcare is taken care of by family members while the food supply and shelter are shared. Should anyone get out of line, threatening the collective balance and harmony, the situation is managed by a group of elders.

For valuable insight into this way of living, you might like to view the television series *Native Wives*. Young women whose lives were basically a mess were placed individually into isolated villages, operating at a third-world subsistence level. Within the first week, every last one of these women experienced a tearful breakdown followed by a joy-filled breakthrough. By being away from all distractions and stopping their harried life, they were able to let go of the stresses they had become accustomed to. The result of this change could be their only ever experience of body systems operating normally. Most of the women also experienced real love and support for the very first time. With the isolation of early learning centers and child care facilities at one end and residential care for the elderly at the other, we are stuck in the middle, isolated behind our fences or in our homes and apartments, spinning on the hamster wheels of our far-too-busy lives.

We are locked into working long hours to make enough money to pay for all of the child and pet care that allow us to work in the first place. Then, of course, there is all of the stuff we are reminded of daily that we need to buy to make us *happy*. More work has to pay for all of those things. As if that isn't enough, there is the added expense of the medical help we now require to manage the sickness generated by this frantic lifestyle. Then there's the media. A few hundred years ago, our ancestors lived in small communities—where change was relatively slow and the news was mostly local. In fact, any news would have come from the neighbors. We then *progressed* to hearing news from the world at the end of the day. As already mentioned in Chapter 5, our televisions used to deliver this with the evening news, which then further *progressed* into our mornings, then regularly throughout our day. Now, thanks to our hand-held devices, there's no need to wait until we get home to watch all of the bad news. We don't have to miss anything. As the old newsroom saying goes, "If it bleeds it leads." So just a couple of clicks away, anywhere, anytime, we can watch the very latest carnage from around the globe. Reports of rape, murder, vehicle pile-ups, extreme weather events, fire, drought, war, famine, disease, violent protests, home invasions, mass shootings, terrorism—it's all on demand in front of us. Added to the stress of exposure to this carnage is knowing that we have no power to influence any of it. Stress without a cure! This lifestyle is one of elevated living.

In order to maintain this pace, we need to push ourselves past our natural body rhythms. For this, we have caffeine, alcohol, sugar, and an ever-increasing array of pharmaceuticals to help us carry on by distancing ourselves from our body's natural warning system. We can't stop because it's all mapped out, and once we step on that wheel we have to keep going. Once we get the mortgage for the house, then pay for the car, boat, holiday, caravan, and the kids' education, we're locked into life in the fast lane. Oh, I nearly forgot about the children's activities. Sport, which used to be recreational even at the highest level, is now seriously competitive and all about winning, including on a child's level. This now requires somewhere near four, or in some cases more, attendances every week at the school level. And then there's martial arts, dance classes, music, and so it goes on, gobbling up any space for unstructured play. We now have two speeds: stressed-out or asleep. Then there's the online gaming and social media, which removes us from communicating with those around us into a distant world of online friends. A friend used to be the person who would be there for you in times of strife. Now "friends" make up the hundreds or possibly thousands of people you may never even meet. The cyber-world contains very little real natural consequence or accountability and the absence of real connection, which opens a huge door to harm. Because this way of living is forced, unhealthy, and counterintuitive, we have to push ourselves into the habit of masking to carry on. Of course, taking care of our exhaustion is seen as a weakness. It flies in the face of being driven to be the best compared to all others. And how much of this do we leave behind when we die? Everything.

## WE REWARD EXTREMISM

In the Western world, we are in love with pressure. I've already written about how our society is based on the belief that winning is the ultimate, bigger is better, regular change is necessary, and possessions and achievements make us happy. We strive for these heady aspirations by overriding the body's natural rhythms. But there is one more blind spot. In order for us to win, someone else must lose. By charging more for less, retailers are trying to win this game, but their customers then need to generate more income, and so it goes on with us chasing our own tails. *Is my house, car, boat, spa pool enough? Are my kids achieving enough? Is my job impressive enough? How many social media followers noticed me today? Is that a line on my face? Must get more Botox and fillers! Being an online influencer, it's essential to pretend that my life is perfect and I am not affected by stress or aging.*

High levels of achievement can represent success and can be a great asset to any community if attained wisely. The problem is, this aspiration to greatness can and does cause us irreparable harm. No one on their deathbed ever said, "I wish I had accumulated more expensive stuff." Our local high school has a big sign inspired by this way of thinking, intentionally positioned right beside the main entrance: a larger-than-life image of the school's four highest-achieving pupils. I wondered at the time what this does, not only to their own perception of work-life balance but to all of the other parents, students, and teachers passing that sign every day. How would it feel to be one of the 600 or so students who could never be the best, no matter how hard they worked? The signboard could easily be replaced with pictures of students who had overcome adversity by thriving against the odds. Aotearoa, New Zealand, currently holds the world record for teenage suicide. We come in second only to Latvia in school bullying and rank thirty-seventh in the world when it comes to adult literacy and numeracy.

Clearly, what we are doing is not working. Mary told me recently that teenagers are the canaries in our coal mine. Before gas detection systems were invented, miners used to take a caged canary into the mine. If there were toxic gases present, the canary would die and the miners would all exit.

In the same week, I listened to a client talking about his high-school-age son—the one I had seen about a year previously for a relatively minor complaint. I remember how full of life and literally bursting with enthusiasm he was. He was super talented and filled with boundless energy, "heading for the top," yet he had gotten into a state of either flat-out or asleep. Every waking moment (including very late in the evenings) he was focused on reaching the next milestone toward greatness. About one year later, when I asked how his son was now, his father paused and then told me quietly that he had become ill. He had begun feeling chronically fatigued and had been diagnosed with possible myalgic encephalomyelitis (ME) and was taking a year off from school and sports in the hope that it would help. A little pressure is healthy, but anything subjected to more sustained pressure than it was designed to handle will at some stage fail, including us! This failure can be subtle at first, but if the warning signs are repeatedly overridden and exposure continues for long enough, the collapse will eventually become catastrophic. I have listened to enough clients describing their own personal experiences of burnout to understand that you can recover, but never fully.

One described life on the other side as having been like a glass that was smashed and super-glued back together. From a distance, it still looked like glass, but on closer inspection, it had many flaws. Apart from it no longer being able to reliably hold liquid, when exposed to more than even the slightest sustained pressure, it would collapse. The client who shared this analogy told me that he always thought he could cope pretty well in his job of managing about seventy-five staff, having been promoted off the tools into the office. He was using alcohol in the evenings, then it increased to sleeping pills, painkillers, and anti-inflammatories daily. "But doesn't everybody do that?" he said. "No, not healthy people," I replied. Then one morning, sitting at his office desk, deciding which pen to pick up became too much, too big a decision! This sudden realization triggered a panic attack, coupled with an uncontrollable outpouring of emotion and tears. A week later he was still bursting into tears many times every day, for at least half an hour each time. In recovery about a month later, he remembered some of the warning signs that burnout was approaching. Those were indications that the light at the end of his tunnel was actually the headlight of an approaching train. Sadly, he had chosen to ignore all the signs. This life pressure, transitional in our minds, accumulates in our bodies. The steadily accumulating nervous energy eventually travels all the way out to the fingers and toes. It's nearly invisible in the rest of the body and becomes much harder to ignore in the hands.

Increased pulling forces on muscles and bones cause them to retract and compress, dehydrating the joints. Most common among females is the very strong link between plantar fasciitis and burnout. The clients I have seen presenting with this symptom could be most accurately described as "full of tension." Usually, it was the result of

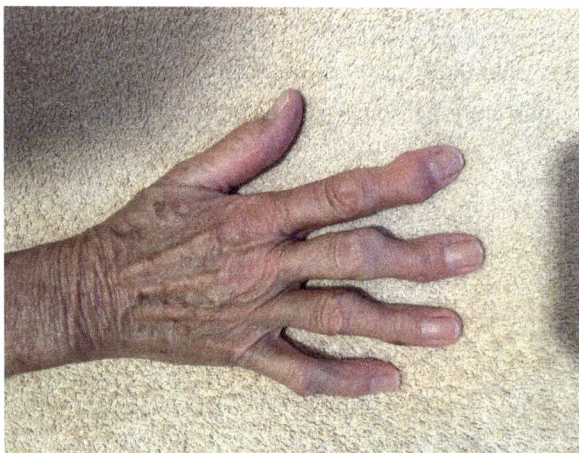

perfectionism or the ridiculous notion of being able to do more than a day's work in a single day.

"I was going along fine until the wheels came off" is a saying that has been used over the years to describe when life stresses get too much for us and our bodies can no longer cope with the load. Please don't try this at home. Any car with a wheel nut removed from each wheel can probably be safely driven slowly to the local dairy once a week. Holding only the driver and staying below 50 kph, there is very little chance of failure. Load the same car with people and luggage and head out onto the open road at 100 kph, and the wheels will very quickly fall off! We are affected by extra loading in a similar way. Whatever inherited genetic weaknesses we are predisposed toward usually tick along undetected until they are amplified by an increase in life pressure. Slight exposure to transitional stress and anxiety is, for the most part, manageable. What can have any of our metaphorical wheels falling off, is a prolonged increase in stress and anxiety.


### MARY

*"My hips have become really sore again, and they are keeping me awake at night like they used to. You got me better, but something must be wrong again because they hurt."*

*"How are your stress levels? Has there been an increase?" I asked.*

*"No, I don't get stressed."*

*Then much later in the session she admitted, "I have just had some people staying at our place for an unusually long time, and it does put me under a lot more pressure. You see, I have to do everything myself."*

By accumulating a residue, we begin each new day with more pressure already onboard than the previous one, and because the deterioration is gradual, we incrementally learn to live with it, just like stopping hearing the planes in the airport analogy.

Tension accumulates inside of us, much like a bucket under a dripping tap. At first, all we notice is a gradual reduction in flexibility

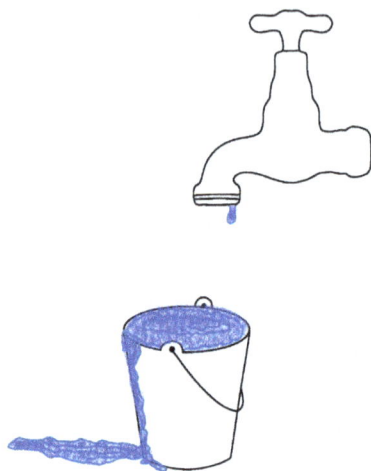

and low-level pain. But as our tension bucket fills, it becomes progressively hard to ignore. Taking medication can provide short-term relief, but the downside is that pain reduction allows us to carry on doing damage. Over time we lose our flexibility, and it becomes progressively more difficult to look over our shoulder or to reach our shoes!

## STRESS CAUSES BODY PAIN

We all know the stress and anxiety are causing the pain, but it's not okay to publicly admit such a dirty little secret, right? More often than not, there is a perfectly logical physical explanation presented. A common scenario I hear is: *"I have a pain in my lower back, which makes it hard to move my right leg. It happened when I got out of the car a week or so ago. Can you help me?"* The rest of our injury-causing story tends to get left out. For example. *"I am suffering from stress and anxiety-related body pain and stiffness. Having inherited a low resistance to conflict situations, I have an ongoing disagreement with yet another work colleague that I just can't resolve. I'm walking on eggshells all day! As a result, I am holding steadily increasing tension throughout my whole body, which is disturbing my sleep. My overall flexibility has reduced to the point where normal functions generate pain. My breathing has become short to the point where I can't even fill my lungs past about 25 percent. The pain is constant, and I have to use large doses of medication to cope. I have been offered cortisone injections and prednisone, but I've read they only mask the problem, may cause harm, and you have to keep getting more. Can you help me?"*

There is nothing to be gained by squeezing the life out of a salt shaker or holding the steering wheel with white knuckles. Both of those things work perfectly well with light pressure. Why do we share this collective elephant in our room? Are we prepared to get sick to maintain this illusion of strength?

We call people and situations a "pain in the neck" or "pain in the arse," but do we really understand the origins of these sayings? Those people and things are what make that part of our body so tight that it begins to break down and send us warning signals in the form of pain. Interactions that *make our blood boil* or *tie our stomach up in knots* actually do that. Why else would we have this age-old language that makes these connections?

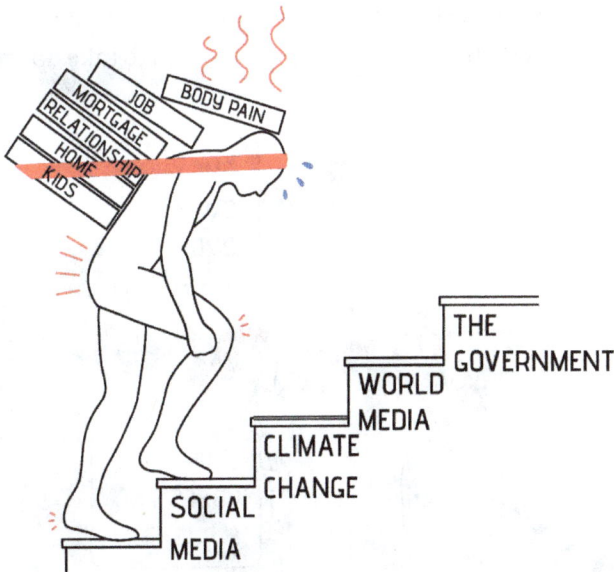

## MARY

*"I was coping, all right. Sure, I was lying awake at night, worrying about what might happen if the interest rates on our mortgage went up a bit more. Then there's the hassle of moving my parents into dementia care. Oh, and we got some enormous bills from the vet, but at least our dog is still alive at age eighteen. Things were going along pretty well, but then my neck and back started to get really sore. My boss is off sick, and her work load has been added to mine until they can find someone new. I was coping with this pretty well until this pain started getting to me. It's in my neck and shoulder, and I have been managing it pretty well with over-the-counter medication. But wouldn't you know it, with my rotten luck, now I've got tennis elbow and my hands are starting to go numb and seize up. Very poor timing. Don't you think?"*

Of course, there is an obvious link here between the stress and the body pain, but we don't want to admit it. All of this stress creates a massive amount of tension, which breaks the body down. If we keep going while under too much pressure, the body eventually fails. It gets progressively tighter and more sore. As one muscle group compacts and loses strength, those still working are forced to take up the strain.

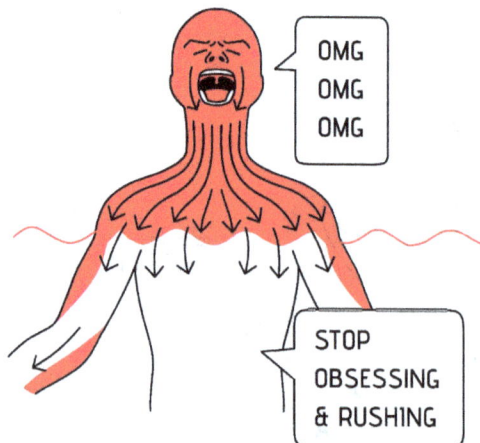

# PUTTING YOUR HAND ON THE HEATER

I have tried all sorts of explanations with clients over the years about the effect of stress on the body, and most did not fully understand it. Then I came up with what I call "putting your hand on the heater." You could attend lectures all week about what it feels like to burn your hand on a heater and still not fully understand. But if the first class on the first day started with you actually burning your hand on a heater, you would be able to go home with a complete understanding. I promise this next simple exercise will not burn you; hopefully, it will convey an all-too-elusive message in an instant.

## STAGE ONE

*Hold out your hand and make a fist. Keep squeezing it shut as tight as you can for about a minute and then quickly open it and have a look at the inside surface. You will see that it has gone pale from the blood having been squeezed out. You will then be able to watch it turn from pale back to its natural color (sustained pressure-related circulation failure and restoration through relaxation).*

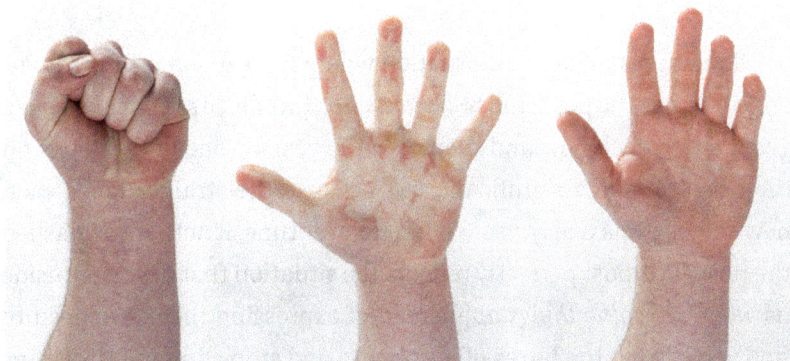

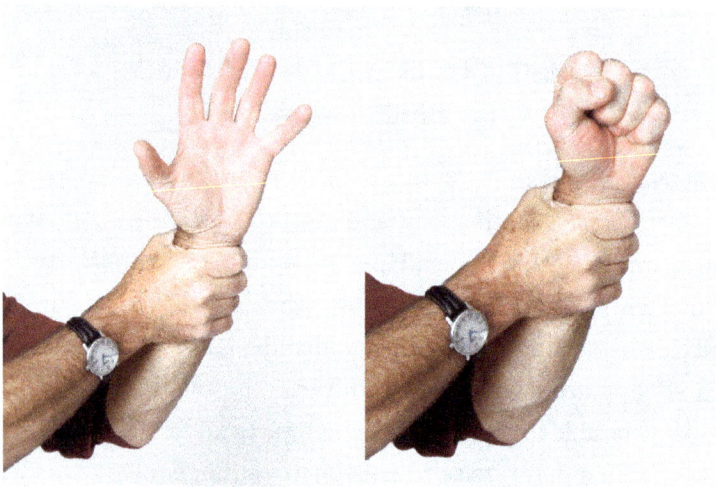

## STAGE 2

*Open and close your left hand while squeezing your left wrist tightly with your right hand. Release your right hand's grip on your wrist while continuing to open and close your left hand (stress-related tension restricts natural body movement, generating pain until released).*

## STAGE 3

*Interlock your fingers and squeeze tightly for about a minute. Then separate and look at how the sides of the fingers are already dented (sustained pressure compacts tissue).*

Sometimes we are in a situation where there is something said or done that has the potential to *wind us up*. This fence strainer has been given a wee click now and then over the years. None of the clicks on their own are very significant, but because the strainer holds each new setting, this one got so wound up over time, it actually squashed the post. This post perfectly reflects the situation that develops inside us when we *bottle things up* instead of expressing them. We need to find ways to get the boxes off our backs and stop climbing the stairs,

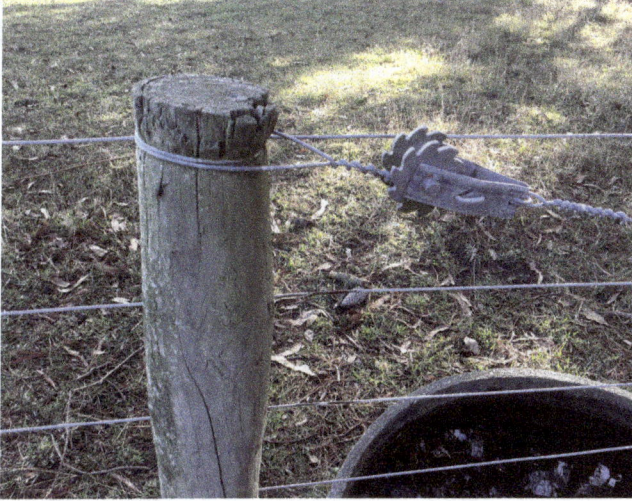

or these muscular clenched fists will continue to spread throughout our bodies.

If you do a search for Polymyalgia Rheumatica, you will find the common translation for this disorder is "many sore, stiff muscles brought on by stress in the over-fifty population." Fibromyalgia is another diagnosis that follows similar patterns. It is listed as a disorder characterized by widespread musculoskeletal pain and is accompanied by fatigue and sleep, memory, and mood issues that may be eased by medication and/or stress reduction. Our bodies do not independently manufacture these diseases. We do this to ourselves. The cause is listed as unknown, but all you need for diagnosis is pain at a total of eighteen recognized locations. The next sketch (overleaf) is designed to give you an idea of a few of the more common dysfunctions that can be caused by the spreading of these pain-filled, movement-restricting metaphorical clenched fists.

This is by no means a complete list, but you may spot something familiar. The fisting compaction of our tissues can cause a lot of breakdowns through direct mechanical pressure, but there is a potentially far more serious side effect, which I call the billabong effect.

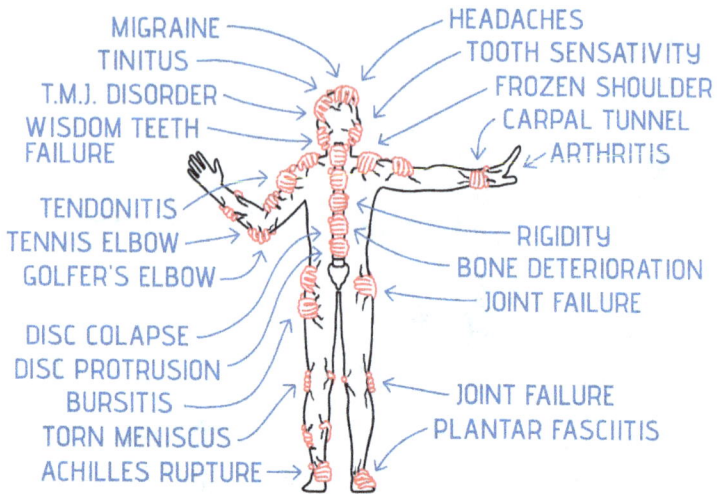

MIGRAINE — HEADACHES
TINITUS — TOOTH SENSATIVITY
T.M.J. DISORDER — FROZEN SHOULDER
WISDOM TEETH — CARPAL TUNNEL
FAILURE — ARTHRITIS

TENDONITIS
TENNIS ELBOW — RIGIDITY
GOLFER'S ELBOW — BONE DETERIORATION
— JOINT FAILURE

DISC COLAPSE
DISC PROTRUSION
BURSITIS — JOINT FAILURE
TORN MENISCUS — PLANTAR FASCIITIS
ACHILLES RUPTURE →

# THE BILLABONG EFFECT

Occasionally a river carves a new path, which can leave a section of the old stream bed isolated. Cut off from the natural flow, these billabongs (Australian aboriginal term) become stagnant, and the water very quickly turns bad. Okay, so this is not a true billabong, but I think this small pond on the left gives a good visual of how stagnation looks. It only took a couple of weeks for the fresh water that was used to fill this pond to go bad. This same scenario is carried out wherever we hold enough stress in our soft tissues to interrupt blood flow. The multiple sore points I have just listed originate wherever our tissues have

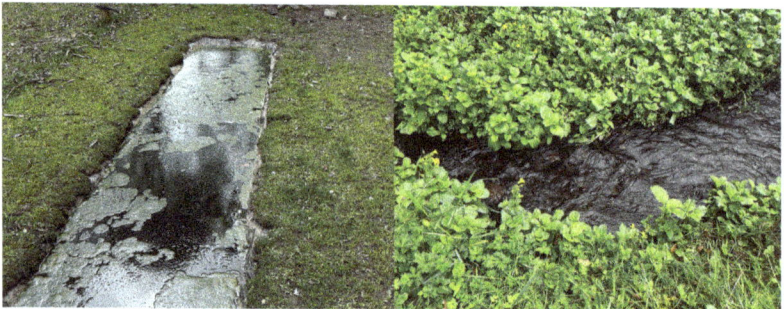

become tight enough to cease functioning normally. Once this blood-starved stagnation occurs, pain is generated to alert us to our body's billabongs. The image on the right is of a spring-fed stream. You can see in an instant the life that fresh flowing water generates.

There are medical procedures available to inject freshened blood into these clenched toxic points, but wouldn't you rather restore your circulation by softening, stretching, and relaxing the tissues? It seems fitting to end this chapter with a few words of wisdom taken from the back of Mainfreight trucks. Sayings that lean into opposing our collective misdirection.

- "Strive not for greatness but to be great."
- "Compete only with who you were yesterday."
- "Shrouds do not have pockets."
- "Doubt your fears, not your dreams."

Chapter 13 is directed toward one of the questions I hear most often: "Why does it really hurt there?"

# STRESS-RELATED HOLDING PATTERNS

## COMMON LANGUAGE

*"I'm holding it all inside."*
*"You are so rigid in you're thinking."*
*"Giving someone a wind up."*

## QUICK FIX

Complacency regarding steadily increasing physical restrictions incrementally reduces our overall ability to move. Some sections of the body become totally immobilized. Doing the mobility tests at the end of this chapter will reveal any limitations that you have grown accustomed to.

## THE HEDGEHOG EFFECT

We all know about the fight-or-flight response, but there is a third option: *freeze*. Under attack, our prehistoric ancestors who were neither fit enough to flee nor strong enough to fight had a third option: Utilizing their *knee-jerk reaction*, they could curl up in a ball like a hedgehog, giving them the best possibility of surviving the attack, albeit a little the worse for wear! Being tightly tucked into the fetal position protects the body's vitals. Do a quick internet search of basic human anatomy and you will see that all of your essential plumbing and wiring runs down the inside of your limbs. We could survive a cut to any of these systems in our extremities because it only feeds a small area, but severing one of your main supply lines would be fatal. The largest veins and arteries are tucked away deep in the body cavity, exiting the legs and arms only toward the inside front of the torso. The bony skull, ribs, spine, and pelvis provide the body with its armor. As the skull drops onto the rib cage, covering the main arteries in the front of the throat, the rib cage closes down onto the pelvis, protecting the vital organs. The limbs wrap tightly against the body and conceal the remaining exposed frontal region and the flanks. Most of what is left exposed is repairable. Painful? Yes. Potentially debilitating and open to infection? Yes. But not imminently life-threatening. This age-old intuitive survival mechanism of body flexions is causing a lot of our present-day pain and discomfort. When we get a really big fright, like when a car backfires or a door suddenly slams, our body is triggered into the freeze flexion. Engaging our survival response, these frights momentarily activate all of our flexors from top to bottom and can be violent enough to lift our feet off the ground. The key here is the word *momentarily*. With any passing danger, predator, or slamming door, once the coast is clear, we are programmed to relax. Everything you have read in the previous chapters has been leading up to the fact that we have lost our sense of safety. Without safety we cannot relax, so all of the muscles that used to momentarily contract us into the freeze position, our flexors, stay a little switched on, sectionally freezing us. What separates us now, is no longer whether or not we hold tension; it is now how much and where we store it. Data from a 2023 National American Institute of Health Survey reported 24.3 percent of the adult population to be living with chronic pain.[1] All of the holding patterns identified in this chapter produce chronic pain. What is crucial to understand is that our body does not initiate any of these responses. They are triggered by the thoughts that we hold.

## MARY

*"You need to fix my body. I've been told that the problem is in my head, but that's bullshit because my head is fine. I just have a frozen shoulder and a friggin tight back. My stupid body hates me. It just needs to shut up and get on with it."*

Mary's body had been sending her head pain signals from a condition that had progressed into a fibromyalgia diagnosis. A very high achiever, running a medium-sized business with her husband and a home with several children, she had become accustomed to a huge amount of daily stress. Her busy lifestyle required her to take her phone to the treatment table. Embodying this very high level of constant arousal is causing an alarming number of us to progressively lose a large portion of our natural ability to move. Body changes brought on by stress occur as we go about our daily lives and happen so slowly that they are barely noticeable. This incremental debilitation reminds me of a story told to me years ago by a counselor. He was explaining how stress invisibly builds in our lives and said that in a similar way it was possible to kill a frog by putting it in cold water and very gradually turning up the heat. Apparently, the changes are so slight that the frog does not notice the temperature rising and eventually dies. I hasten to add that I have never done this, and neither should anyone. Thanks, though, to this horrific example, I better understood how we are able to subtly accumulate stress-related tension until our condition becomes chronic. What is starting in our minds and ending up in our bodies does not apply to just a few of us. It's all too easy to think that no one else is affected in this way, but to some degree we all are. What can seem individual and isolating has actually become a non-viral pandemic. I have named some of our favorite places to hold a bit of tension.

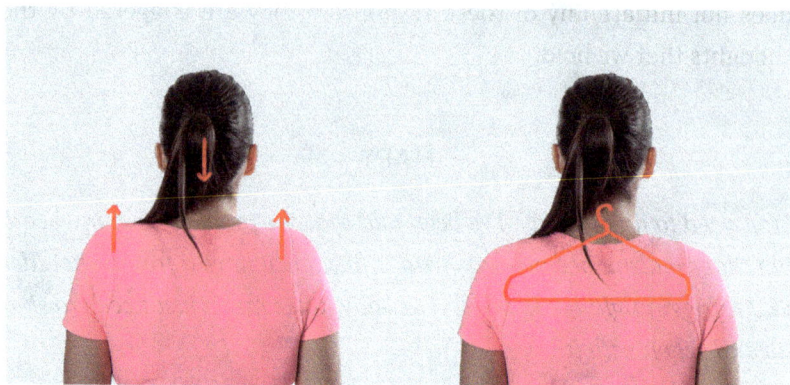

# TURTLE NECK

## MARY

"*People tell me that when I am doing the school timetables every year, it's the same. It's a massive job and has to be done on time, in addition to my normal full workload. My head starts pulling in and my shoulders lift up with all of the stress. My colleagues call it my turtle neck.*"

The turtle neck is probably the most common form of stress-related holding. Sitting for prolonged periods hunched over a keyboard will not produce this body freeze on its own. What does the damage is the stress-response muscle flexion between the shoulders and neck. As we sit working hard, while "stressing out," we engage the survival muscle flexions that are used to protect the front of our throat from attack. This age-old stress response draws the shoulders up and closes the head down and forward. Do this for long enough and often enough and your muscles will lock you short, holding this neck scrunch like a freeze-frame.

# THE COAT HANGER

Imagine you could glue a coat hanger across your upper back and neck and not have it shift or bend as your body moves. There is no shortening of the neck or visible hunching of the shoulders, but the whole area is rigid. It is most easily noticeable in joggers. Their arms swing forward and back with nothing moving in between. Your arms do not reach very far by themselves and need your shoulders' mobility to complete gross movements.

*Stand with your arms hanging loosely beside your body, then raise one up to level. It makes no difference whether you did this to the side or out in front of you. What you have just done is raise your arm to the limit of what I call your first shoulder joint's travel. The muscles that do this are across what is commonly known as your shoulder joint. Because of this, they are relatively near the top of your arm. Now continue raising your arm until it will not go up any farther. This action utilizes what I call the second shoulder joint. To access this second ninety degrees of travel, your shoulder blade rotates, taking your outstretched arm up to vertical. If you do have a "coat hanger" across your upper body, your shoulder blade will not rotate, and your arm will not extend far past horizontal.*

## THE TEDDY BEAR

A more advanced level of the coat hanger is the teddy bear. This immobilizes the entire torso. The teddy bears among us usually don't jog

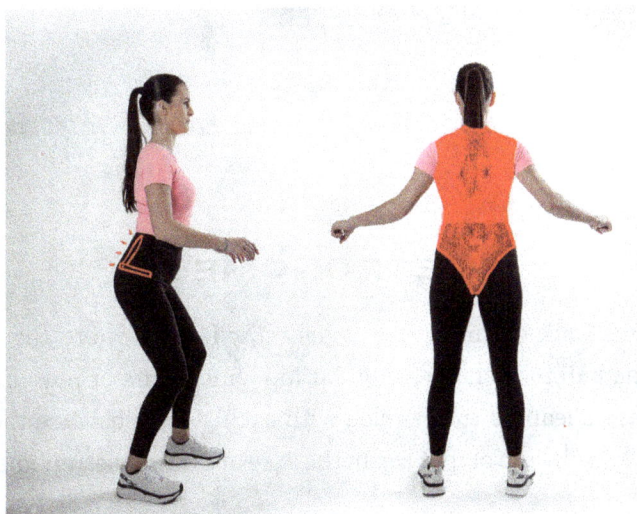

because of the jarring. Cycling is still an option as the stiffened body can be motionless, supported by the bike seat. When walking, teddy bears tend to swing their arms awkwardly from side to side, across, and in front of themselves to compensate for the total lack of body mobility.

## THE RUSTY POCKETKNIFE

Rusty pocket knives dread sitting even though it doesn't hurt. What gets them is knowing the pain they will have to go through to get up again. With pelvic and lower back joints dehydrated and stiffened, this lower section of the spine gradually creeps and locks forward with the micromovements of sitting for a long time. Trying to stand up again instantly pressurizes this locked-forward area, which then means the bearer has to take those agonizing steps to return to *almost vertical.* The more severe cases, having lost all hope of standing up straight again, adopt the habit of walking with their hands locked behind their backs in an attempt to counterbalance their forward body weight.

### PETER

*"People keep telling me to stand up straight, but it hurts to do that. So I stay a little forward with my hands behind my back. I suppose that is making it worse."*

## METRONOMES

When we walk normally, our bodies stay fairly close to the center. With the half metronome, singular hip joint failure or muscle weakness has us leaning to that side with each step to balance the body weight over the top of that leg. In the case of the full metronome, there is a hip deterioration or muscle weakness on both sides, which causes the body to sway sideways in the direction of the fault with every step.

## THE IRONING BOARD

With every new client, I do a total-body response test to check how widespread the restrictions are. If wiggling the feet from side to side also moves the head, their body tension is complete, hence the name. This absolute tension can be overwhelming and very difficult to accept. I have yet to find a single ironing board that admits their totally rigid state. This level of total static strain eventually causes tendonitis and bursitis.

## TENDONITIS & BURSITIS

### MARY

*"I've been diagnosed with gluteal insertional tendonitis but the strange thing is I don't remember any accident that might have caused it."*

Mary had gathered tension throughout the whole lower to mid-section of her body. Most of her muscles felt more like blocks of wood than soft tissue. Diagnoses ending in "itis" describe inflamed tissue. And, yes, her gluteal tendons were indeed running red-hot. Not through any fault of their own, they were generating pain, alerting her to the constant strain. That's why I prefer to call it *"tendon tightis."* This is a perfect example of what Dr. Jo talked about when diagnosing body-pain issues while looking through a microlens. Anything done to silence the tendon's alarms locally would have allowed Mary's overall condition to stay constant, under her radar, or further deteriorate. Probably to the detriment of the hip joints, which under this much constant pressure would inevitably fail. This same scenario applies to bursitis. A bursar is a fluid-filled tissue bubble that provides

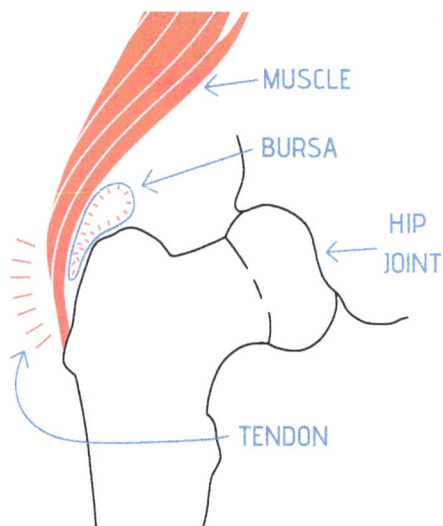

cushioning anywhere tendons can rub against bones. They swell and get painfully inflamed under sustained pressure. The solution is the same for both: Leave the symptomatic tendons and bursas alone and eliminate the overarching life and body tensions.

## USE IT OR LOSE IT

The following drawing depicts the shrinking of our upper body's physical ability that can limit our movements as we age. This can happen so gradually over time that we barely notice the changes. All that is required for this range-of-motion decay to begin is to stop using the end range of any movement.

The regular gross weight-bearing movements of our normal daily activities used to keep us mobile. Walking to the clothesline, washing basket in hand, reaching up and down to hang the clothes, swinging the axe repeatedly, stacking away the wood. Physical tasks like these kept all of our moving parts fully functional. Now all we have to do is pop it in the machine and push a button or switch.

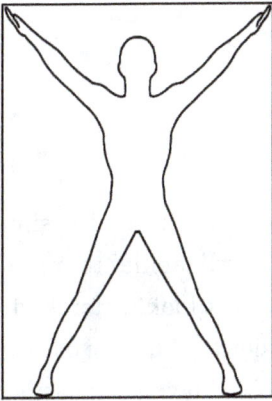 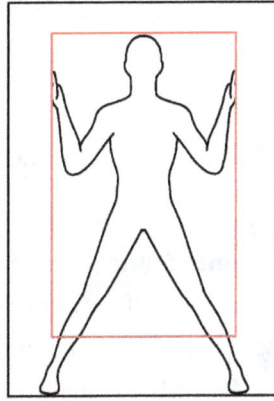

# POTENTIAL  REALITY

Before the days of professional sporting teams, the strength and endurance of the Westland Rugby League players was legendary. They were supremely fit and strong because they shoveled coal all day, every working day. Now players live at the gym to achieve this same level of strength and fitness, which is what we all need to do more of as machines have replaced many tasks. The worst thing we can do is to stop trying. An alarming number of us have let go of some of the most basic of our abilities, like getting down on the floor and back up again. It is incredibly unsafe to be unable to get up once you have fallen down. I'm not going to name the age at which this inability usually kicks in, but let's just say that if you're getting close to the twilight years, you need to get down and lie flat on the floor and then get right back up again without holding on to the furniture. Once you have done that, repeat using the side that is more diffi-cult. Do this every day. Then, if you do have a fall, you won't have to wait there for hours, or possibly several days, until someone finds you. Reaching up and bending over needs to be done regularly too. In fact, all of our natural movements require regular attention to ensure their survival. The restrictions that limit our movements tend to freeze our thinking as well.

## POTENTIAL FOR IMPROVEMENT

The following measurements are designed as a fairly simple checklist, or "warrant of fitness," for our overall ability to move as nature intended. The range of movement you are looking for is what is commonly accepted as "normal" (the majority). Some of us are built with restrictions and others are hypermobile. If you can easily bend your thumb back and bring it to rest against the side of your wrist you either have a dislocated thumb or some degree of hypermobility. There are some extremely hypermobile people who can be seen at the circus folding their body into a small glass box. Then there are those of us who must have been put together on a day when there were a few extra bits lying around in the factory. Ending up with a couple of added ribs or an extra vertebra or two does not make a lot of difference. The real test for each one of us is whether or not anything negatively impacts our daily life. For a quick heads-up on how much more functional you could be, you may like to take a few minutes to go through this list. Please exercise care when attempting any of these tests, and never push into pain. If anything hurts, don't do it.

- TOUCH YOUR TOES
    *Stand up with your knees locked, or sit on the floor with your legs flat, and attempt to touch your toes. Please don't blame your hamstring for any lack of travel. Most people who do don't realize the problem is actually their rigid back.*

- BODY TURN
    *Seated, fold your arms and rotate your upper body through ninety degrees left, then right.*

- HANDS HIGH

  *Reach up with both hands at once as if trying to touch the ceiling. Keep going until they won't extend any farther. If anything feels tight or the arms are not parallel and straight up, there is room for improvement.*

- BEHIND BACK

  *Reach down and back with one hand at a time to touch the bottom edge of your opposite shoulder blade with your fingertips.*

- PULLING YOUR LEG

  *Lying on your back, leave one leg out flat and, with fingers locked together, clasp your other knee and pull it toward your chest. Free of any static restrictions, your held leg will come to rest on the side of your chest without the relaxed leg moving.*

- CROUCH UNSUPPORTED, HEELS ON THE FLOOR

  *It might be a good idea to hold onto a table or desk if you are doing this for the first time as you may need some help to get vertical again. Standing with your feet directly below your hips, get into a crouched position without lifting either of your heels off the floor. The goal is to comfortably balance unsupported in the crouched position with the upper leg horizontal or lower.*

- THE UNDIES TEST

  *Holding a pair of undies with both hands, put them on without letting go.*

- FOREARM MUSCLES

  *Hold your straight arm out in front of you, level with your shoulder, and press your hand flat against the wall. Then repeat using the back of your hand. Anything less than a ninety-degree angle at the wrists indicates room for improvement.*

This is by no means a complete full-body checklist, but these will have already given you a pretty good heads-up on how much natural mobility you have or may have lost.

## PETER

*Peter's "teddy bear" torso saw him literally losing his grip on what had been a very impressive stint at the top of club-level golf. With overall mobility reduced to around 50 percent and constant back pain that often became acute, he was desperately seeking a solution. Predictably, with his pelvis the full 2.5 centimeters out of whack, Peter responded well to treatment. So well, in fact, that on arrival at his fifth appointment, he proudly announced that he was now "bombing the ball." Getting the same distance into the wind that had only been achievable with a tailwind, he had seen the head of his golf club at the end of his swing for the first time ever! His golfing partner had commented that his swing was suddenly looking the best he had seen it and asked how he had achieved that in such a short space of time.*

# CHAPTER 14

# COMPACTION

## COMMON LANGUAGE

*"I was petrified."*
*"She's the rock in our family."*
*"Always had to keep my guard up."*

## QUICK FIX

Stress-induced muscle compaction, strangling healthy tissue, and reducing both strength and mobility can be remediated. Refer to repairs and maintenance chapter for self-treatment suggestions.

Have you ever wondered what makes those painful little knots that sit on your shoulders? You know, the ones that see you heading off to your massage therapist? These tight sore points aren't just restricted to the shoulders; they can develop anywhere there is a muscle. They are not sore because of a fault in the tissue; they are simply letting you know they are too tightly bound. Every part of you is enmeshed in an extremely thin, organic version of carbon fiber mesh called *fascia*. This covering is so well distributed around us that if the rest of what our bodies are made of could somehow be whisked away, we would still be recognizable by a mesh-like version of ourselves. It's this fascia that does the binding. At the cellular level, each muscle is made up of clusters of controllable pistons, and it's these that get stuck.

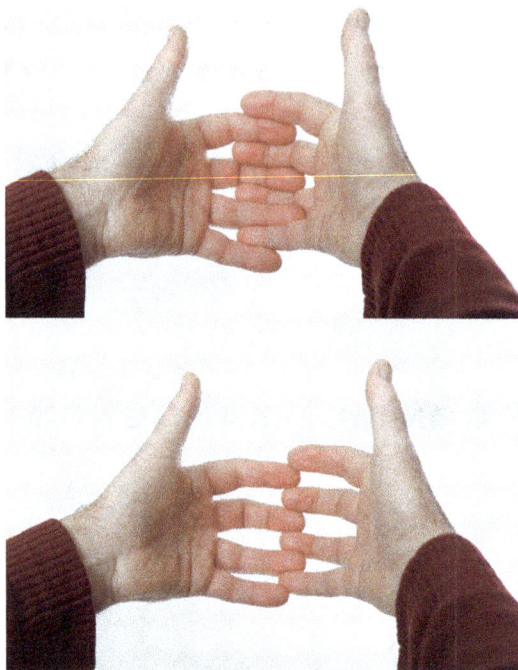

*To get a visual of how muscles behave at the microscopic level, bring your hands together, palms facing you, and slide your interlocked fingers in and out.*

These cells are soft, and without some kind of support wrapped around them, they would easily rupture under pressure, a bit like an egg without the shell. Undisturbed, fascia is tough, light, and thin enough to support all of these parts without getting in the way. This sheathing covers individual cells, bundles of cells, bundles of bundles, and then again over each muscle.

As with most things in life, there are positives and negatives. Yes, facial tissue is incredibly strong and essential when it comes to holding things together, but this strength also makes it very effective at binding. Muscles release once a stimulus is removed; fascia does not. Disturbed for long enough by our nervous energy, fascia shrinks and hardens, strangling our muscles. This vice-like squeeze makes it hard for the affected sections of the muscle to move and more difficult for the circulation to enter and leave. It is this mechanism that can render an otherwise strong muscle group as weak as a kitten.

## WEAK AS A KITTEN

This is how the tension in our lives becomes mirrored in our bodies. The steadily increasing pressure shrinks and shuts down section after section until the muscle is so tightly bound that it is shortened and locked. With reduced energy supply and a steadily reducing number of cells able to move, the muscles are progressively weakened and become an injury waiting to happen. A completely functional muscle is very difficult to tear, but shut down a major section and it's only a matter of time. Most of us would fail to rip a whole ream of printer paper, but divide off about ten percent and you can tear them straight through. This is how our reduced-capacity compacted muscles rupture. Not wanting to display any sign of weakness and with up to 95 percent of the available muscle fibers ineffective, we take a few meds to dull the pain and carry on, then wonder why damage has been done.

## FULLY OPERATIONAL

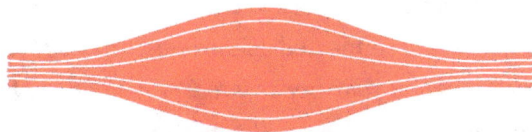

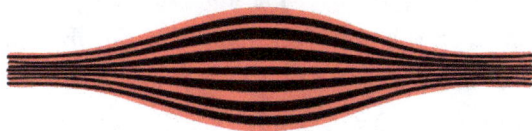

## LESS THAN 50%

*To feel compacted tissue on yourself, place your hand around your forearm with your thumb pointing to your elbow. Gently dig the tip of your thumb into the muscles. Holding a slight pressure and moving your thumb across and back, you will find a muscle or two that feels firmer than the rest and a bit tender. Tinnitus sufferers will be able to easily locate some compacted tissue in their jaw muscles by placing the fingertips of both hands at the rear of both cheeks and gliding them horizontally forward and back. Any bumpy, tender compacted muscles will be more than obvious.*

## LOSING OUR GRIP

If you find yourself reaching for a special tool to help you open the gherkins, or you have a tendency to turn an ankle, you are more than likely suffering from compaction. Just like movement restrictions, it's common to accept these progressive muscle weaknesses as a part of the natural aging process. But if compaction is the cause, and it usually is, they simply require freeing up. Restore them and you will soon be the one that gets handed the jars to open.

Your hands need to have huge muscles strong enough to clamp onto a jungle gym and hold your entire body weight off the ground. Your feet need just as much strength in the opposite direction as they support your body against gravity and propel you forward. Muscles this big would more than double the size of your hands and feet, rendering them useless. So, in a bit of very clever engineering, the muscles were placed past the ankle and wrist and are connected using a series of long tendons.

*Place a firm hold on your upper forearm with one hand while wiggling your other hand and fingers. The movement you can feel is in the muscles that need to be freed. It's the same scenario for your feet. Place another firm hold on your lower leg, about halfway from ankle to knee. Wiggle your toes and then wiggle your whole foot. Neither of these holds will generate any discomfort in healthy limbs, so anywhere you feel pain, once treated, will unlock its true potential.*

Like it or not, these compacted tissues are your stress barometers. As life's pressures ramp up, so does the tension and rigidity. Remember Chapter 4, A State of Unrest, where I wrote about what your body will do to get your attention?

- *There are groupings of cells on every muscle whose job is to generate enough pain to alert you when latent tension has accumulated.*
- *There is no other reason for these knotty, potentially painful alarming points to be there.*
- *The only thing that ever makes these points generate pain signals is sustained overload.*
- *This overloading can be postural or overuse, but in 99 percent of the people I treat, the original cause is emotional, which produces overstimulation combined with lack of movement.*

I know, there I go harping on about stress again, but this list contains one of the most significant messages in the whole book. The solution for all muscles compacted by this buildup of nervous energy is the same: release! They are not damaged, only trapped. There are two very effective techniques to self-treat these problem areas: the pin and stretch, and the trap and wiggle.

## PIN AND STRETCH

If you attempt to stretch out any trapped muscle over its entire length, you run the risk of damaging the muscle, tendons, or the attachments. It could also be unbearably painful. But by pinning only one relatively small part of the affected muscle, the stretch that follows can be concentrated into just that spot being treated. Once released, the point of contact can be moved along in stages one section at a time until the whole muscle is freed. Our forearms are probably the easiest area to self-treat in this way.

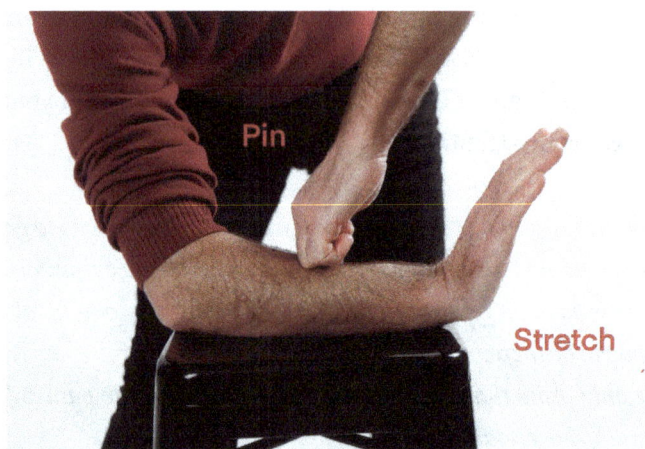

*Lay one forearm parallel with your body on a hard surface with the hand, palm down, past the edge. Next, make a fist with your other hand and bring the knuckles, facing the stationary elbow, down slowly but firmly onto the resting forearm just above the wrist.*

*Dig your knuckles in while raising the fingers of the other hand. Keep the knuckles held firmly against the tissues while slowly bringing the resting hand back down. You will feel the initial pain from the pinning followed by the release once the stretch is complete. Repeat in knuckle-width stages all the way to your elbow.*

## TRAP AND WIGGLE

This is a similar technique to pin and stretch, but this time your focus is only on the most painful spot on any given muscle.

*Rest your thumb in line with your forearm while gently clamping the outside with your fingers. Search around until you have located the most tender spot, and hold it at a pressure that feels uncomfortable. Next, wave your free wrist forward and backward until the pain under your fingers reduces to about half.*

You can successfully treat any muscular pressure point in this way. All you have to do is locate and trap the most painful spot and then

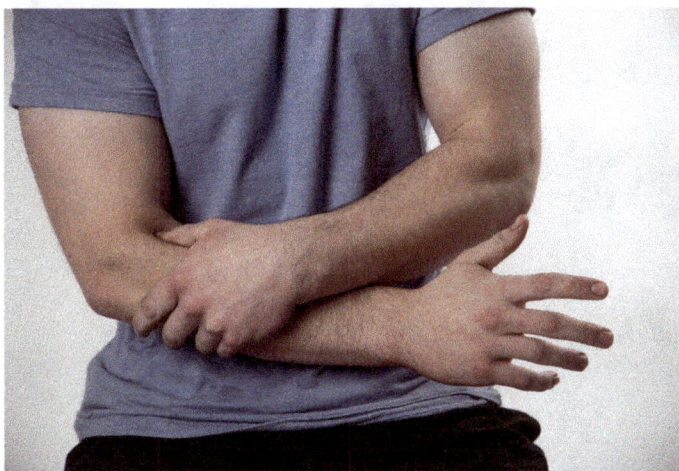

figure out how to get the muscle you have selected to move. An easy one to begin with is your jaw. You can locate the sore spots by pressing your fingers into both sides at once just below your cheekbones, then treat them by opening and closing your mouth. If you find compaction in your jaw muscles, you probably also have a condition called tinnitus.

## TINNITUS

If you suffer from this debilitating condition, you will probably know that the cause is still a mystery. The hissing sizzling sound is generated by compaction. Compacted muscles generate static once compressed. This sound goes under our radar around the rest of our bodies, but those closest to our ears, we can hear. There are several muscle groups close enough to the ears to cause tinnitus once compacted. Probably the most obvious are the ones that work the jaw and at the back of the neck. It's a good thing that our ears are so far away from our tightly compacted back muscles because the static generated there would be unbearable.

*Place a couple of iceblock or chopsticks between your back teeth. Close your jaw firmly, squeezing the wood and releasing it while monitor-*

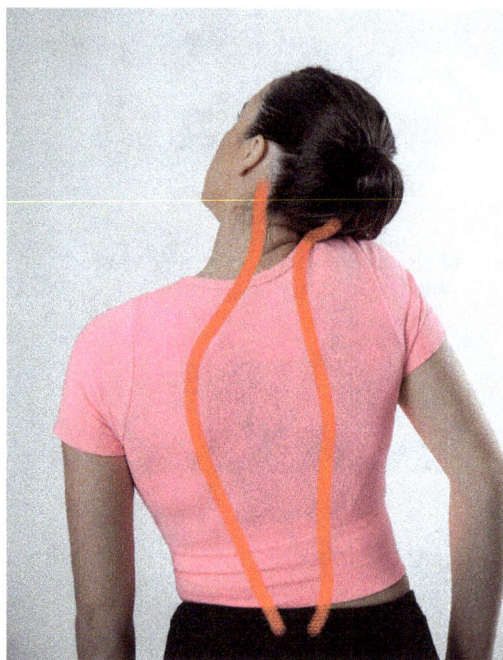

*ing the ringing in your ears. Next, extend your jaw as far forward as you can and then back again. Finally, squeeze the back of your head against one raised shoulder while turning your head away. Any alteration in your tinnitus pitch or intensity indicates that you have located a part of the problem.*

You could prevent compaction from getting re-established in your body by eliminating most of the stress from your life, but this might require you to move to a monastery. In order to avoid compacted tissues becoming a major problem while remaining immersed in our crazy-making society, your body will require regular maintenance, and your mind will need tools to insulate your body from what it has to cope with every day. Stressful situations do not build compaction; our reaction to them does. Find a way to start incorporating micropauses and functional breathing into every day. The tools presented here will keep your mind more relaxed, which of course keeps your body more relaxed. To resolve any already compacted tissue, choose a treatment modality, or several, that work for you.

We can ignore significant levels of pain generated by compaction as we distract ourselves by rushing around throughout the day. But our steadily deteriorating physical state becomes impossible to ignore when we try to sleep.

# CHAPTER 15

# IT'S NEVER THE BED OR PILLOW

## COMMON LANGUAGE

*"You're so full of it!"*
*"I wouldn't trust him. He couldn't lie straight in bed."*
*"That's a bit of a sore point."*

## QUICK FIX

Luxurious bedding feels lovely, costs a lot, and can mask body pain and rigidity in the short term. Shift your focus and your expenditure into finding solutions for your pain and dysfunction rather than accommodating the irritations. Identifying and resolving any chronic pains will assure that you are more comfortable, regardless of your bedding. Adopting the *almost tummy-down* sleep position may help while your condition is improving.

Getting the right amount of sleep is crucial for both mental and physical health. A busy brain can make getting a good night's sleep impossible. By rushing around all day under pressure, we put our true feelings and thoughts on hold. Then we lie down at the end of the day to sleep, wondering why we can't doze off. All of the stuff that has been building up, trying to get our attention all day, is suddenly in plain view. Just like the snowman in the glass dome, we know that all we have to do to pretend he is not there is to keep shaking. But when we lie down and sit the container on the bedside cabinet, slowly but surely all of the snow settles to the bottom and . . . there he is! Not a smiling, carrot-nosed snowman. Because of all our worry and rushing, this snowman is probably red with a long, pointy tail holding a three-pronged spear.

The other sleep stealer is underlying body pain. A neck, shoulder, or hip that's a bit sore during the day can be tolerated for a surprisingly long time because we get distracted. But try sleeping and it's *in your face*. Carrying unresolved body pains and restrictions severely limits not only our sleeping positions but our overall comfort, restricting the amount of sleep we get. Why is this? Because the issues are stuck in our tissues.

## GETTING COMFORTABLE

If your emotional batteries (hip flexors) are partly charged up, your back will constantly ache, and you will have to sleep with your legs bent to make the pain go away. This works because you are reducing the tractional pressure. If your hip flexors are fully charged, you will need a pillow between your knees as well because the inflammation and tension will have migrated into your hips. This also means you will have to keep your legs just as bent when you stand. After all, standing is the vertical version of lying down. The reason the standing image looks a bit strange is that the lying-down image has been rotated up to show how you would have to stand with hip flexors this painfully shortened.

You will more than likely be forced into avoiding the more painful of the two hip positions by rolling to the other side. But body pain progresses diagonally from one hip into the opposite shoulder, so that rules out getting settled on the other side too. So, there you lie, wide

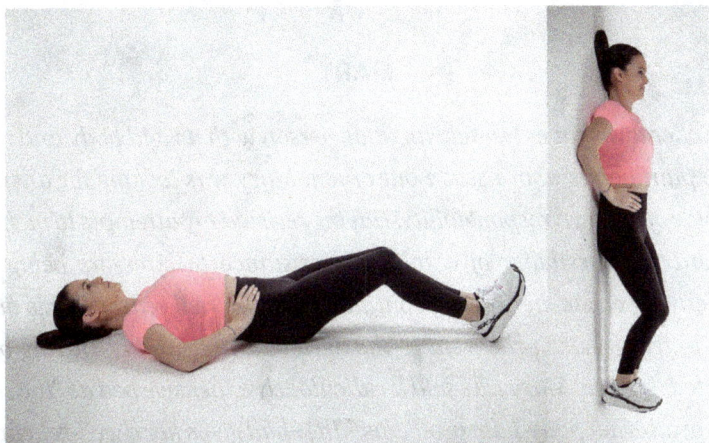

awake, staring at the ceiling, forced onto your back with your bent legs, supported by a pillow, with your neck beginning to ache when it dawns on you . . . *Anyplace on my body that comes into contact with the bed or pillow hurts, what I need is a new bed!.* Should you go shopping for new bedding and pillows? Beware: Softer, more supportive bedding does nothing to improve body pain or stiffness; it simply masks symptoms. Shopping for the perfect sleep with anything less than the perfect body makes you a sitting duck for retailers. Referring again to the same picture, you actually do not need a pillow when you are lying on your back. I know this flies in the face of what we have been doing for millennia, but if you choose to sleep with your head resting on a pillow it is held forward and you are ruining your posture while you sleep. Take a look from the side at anyone with perfect posture and you will notice their head in a straight line with the back of their shoulders and their bottom. Have another look, this time from the front, and you will see the real reason we need pillows. There is a large gap between the head and the side of the shoulder that needs to be filled to keep the neck straight. So keep your pillow handy to use only when lying on your side. (If your posture is poor, you will need to gradually reduce the pillow thickness over time to achieve this.)

## MARY

*This client was an extremely anxious person with a rigid body and mul-
tiple pain points above seven out of ten. Mary was looking for answers
outside of her own responsibility. Having resisted my attempts to inch her
toward the possibility of a lowered resistance to stressors being the
underlying cause, her search continued for the "real reason." This quest
was unfruitful until she went to the agricultural field day. Having been
spotted limping, Mary was sold a ridiculously expensive bed as "the solution to all of her body-pain problems." They had given her a well-rehearsed
rundown on what "this bed could do for her." With full-body massagers,
toppers designed for astronauts, sections that tilt and fold, they all
promised to bring her into the best position for the "optimum sleeping
experience." Of course, the whole setup was recommended by health
professionals. The deal was then sealed by telling her that because her
foot would sometimes go numb, she needed to go for the ultimate pack-
age, which included the leg-raising section. I quote the title of Jeremy
Clarkson's book, "Seriously?"*

A healthy, relaxed, pliable body can sleep pretty much anywhere.
If body pain has you tossing and turning, it's because something internal needs attention. Your body is trying to tell you that it's not in a
healthy state. You should be able to poke yourself pretty much anywhere firmly with your thumb (except in the eye) and feel nothing
but pressure. The other thing essential for a restful night's sleep is
flexibility.

*Sit up straight and tilt your head (ear toward your shoulder) to one
side and then the other, seeing how close to 45 degrees away from the
center you get. Next, with your mouth closed, put your chin to your chest
in a pain-free way and then move it backward to 70 degrees. Lastly, do a
rotation. Be careful to keep your shoulders still. Can your chin come to
rest over the top of your shoulder on either side?*

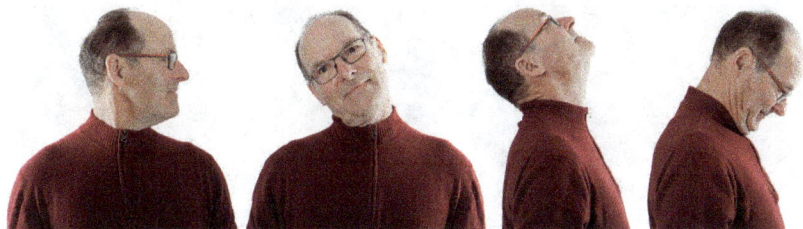

All that you should ever feel is the tissue coming to the end of its natural travel and then stopping pain-free. Don't be too surprised or concerned to score an epic fail here as limitations are common and usually treatable. If it's your pillow you have been having trouble with, you probably have what I call a pencil neck.

## PENCIL NECK

Our necks are potentially strong and very bendy, so why would they need a special pillow to rest them at that exact height through the night? The simplest way I've found to demonstrate what goes wrong with our necks and pillows is with a glue gun stick, a pencil, and a kitchen sponge.

*Place one end of the glue stick on a flat surface and the other on a piece of sponge. By pressing on the middle of the shaft, you will see that the glue stick bends downward and makes little or no impression because it has a full range of flexibility. Next, do the same experiment, but this time using the pencil, demonstrating the small, localized pressurizing contact points generated by rigidity.*

Yes, I know you've already figured out what is going to happen, but it really helps to actually feel and see the difference. Of course, the pencil collapses the makeshift pillow. If you look closely, you will see the tip digging into the towel. Of course, if that were you, it would hurt at those points where it makes contact. If you have a glue gun glue stick type of neck, you could sleep comfortably on just about

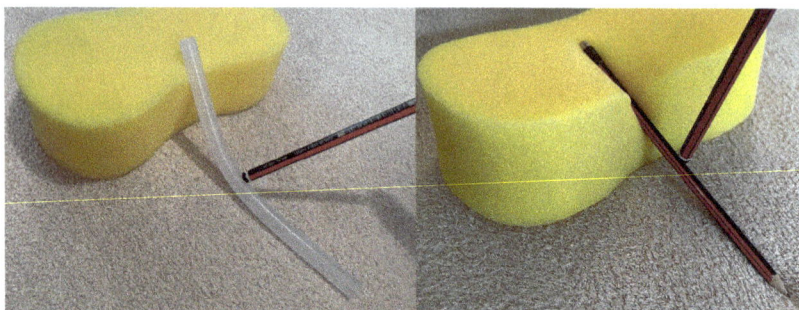

anything, but if you have more like a pencil neck you would still feel some level of discomfort, even on the most elaborate setup.

## MARY

*"I have seven different pillows beside my bed. Each one is good for about three hours, then the agony returning to my shoulder and down my arm forces me to change again to a slightly lower or higher one." Six months later she reported back: "I am desperate! I've bought two more pillows at a stupid price. One was two hundred dollars, and they are both no good!"*

The problem with having an inflexible body is that our weight is no longer evenly distributed along the whole system. A relaxed, pliable body easily follows contours. Rigidity focuses body weight pressure right onto those few mattress and pillow contacting body points that are already sore. This applies equally to wherever it hurts already: head, neck, back, hips, shoulders, arms, and knees. Even one sore toe can keep you awake with the pressure of one just sheet!

The other problem you will be faced with if you buy specialized bedding to manage your dysfunction is that you are trapped at home. Short of taking it all with you, there is no way to guarantee the same standard, even at the top end of accommodation alternatives. This means no school camps, no staying over with friends, no holidays in hotels. "Special" pillows can cost as much as $400 each and beds more than $20,000. So how can we become cozy, restful, and

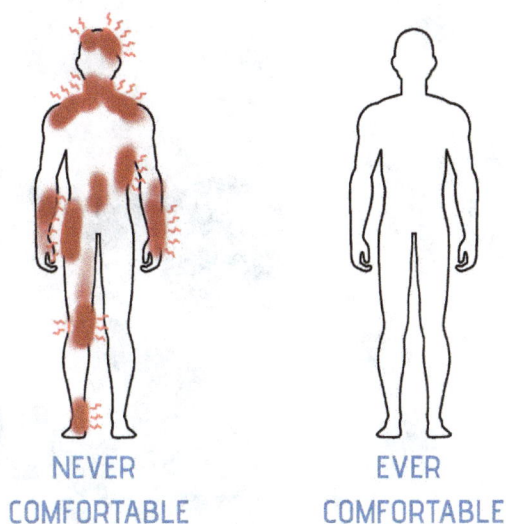

NEVER
COMFORTABLE

EVER
COMFORTABLE

snug? These three words are a far cry from *comfort*, which means to soothe, console, or sympathize. We all know on some level that the trouble really is in our bodies because we have, admit it or not, felt the slow decline over a number of years, all the while convincing ourselves that "it's really not all that bad." Inevitably, it gets to the point where it really is bad enough, and we can no longer ignore it. The truth of the matter is that pencils and stiffened, sore bodies don't bend. The simple answer is to find ways to resolve the issues that are causing all of this discomfort in the first place. Whether you choose lifestyle changes, exercise, yoga, pilates, tai chi, treatments, visiting one of those stress-busting setups where you pay to smash stuff, or a combination of all seven, you must change something. A full recovery can and usually does take a while. In order to get some sleep in the meantime, try lying *almost* tummy down.

## ALMOST TUMMY DOWN

This almost side-lying sleeping position is a modified version of the recovery position.

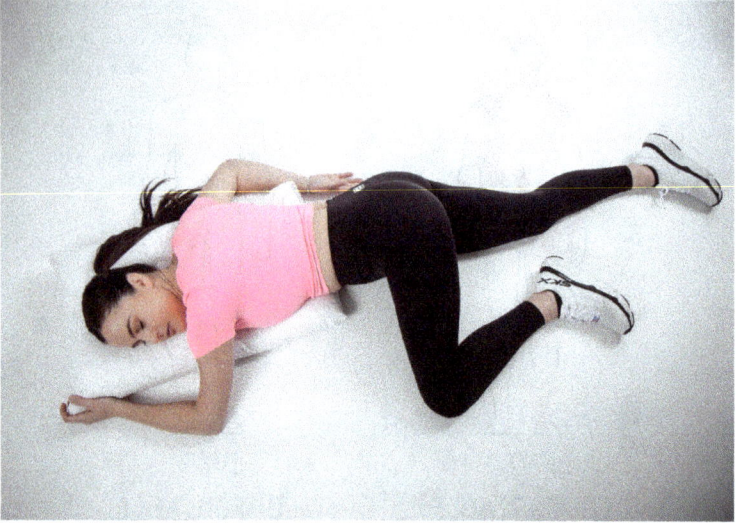

You will find it takes most of the pressure off those sore points.

*Rest your upper body on a pillow, and place your underside arm behind you. I know you think straight away that your arm will go numb, but it won't. In fact, it is the key to making this position work. A slight alteration is to lie on your side as before while bringing your pillow down against your chest and mid-body. While hugging it toward you with your free arm, rest your head on the bit of pillow left at the top. Now straighten the leg closest to the mattress, bend the other one, and...shizam, a better sleep! For extreme dysfunction, add another pillow under your bent leg. This is a pain and stiffness management position, but you may decide to adopt it as your new go-to sleep position.*

### MARY

*"I used to toss and turn for hours at a time, trying to get to sleep, when it dawned on me that this was stressing me even more. One night I lay there and stopped trying, and wouldn't you know it, I went to sleep. Now I tell myself that it's okay if I don't sleep straight away, and it really helps me to relax enough to doze off."*

## DARKNESS

"It was pitch black. You couldn't see your hand in front of your face." We are progressively eradicating this natural total darkness. Satellite images now show what used to be the dark side of our planet, increasingly lit up. Lighting inside our buildings, on our bridges and piers, street lighting, and now skyscrapers that glow, are systematically removing what used to be nighttime. We can block this artificial light out with heavy blackout curtains sealed against the wall but that creates another problem, the absence of gradual transition. The twilight zone has all but disappeared from our planet. This softened shifting in nature from morning to night and back to morning again that takes its own time has been replaced by our light switches and devices, hand-held or not, that are either on or off. These sudden evening flicks from light to dark and then back to light again in the morning create yet another urgency in our increasingly unrested lives. It really is worth a trip into the wilderness to experience the effortless unfurling that happens at the core of your being, as you watch total darkness unhurriedly envelop the land. Then your mind and body, exposed to these gradually transitioning illumination cycles, can truly understand that nighttime is the right time for slowing down and sleeping. There is another natural lesson available to all who choose to experience the dawn chorus as the birds sing their welcome to the slowly rising sun.

## SLEEP APNEA

This diagnosis is now reaching epidemic proportions. A steadily increasing number of us are now using a machine to help us to do one of our most natural bodily functions, sleeping! Before you accept any sleep apnea diagnosis, test yourself. Do you have pain-free, normal mobility? Are you doing thirty minutes of aerobic exercise three times every week that makes you puff? Are you using your diaphragm for breathing? Are you medicating for body pain? Honestly, are you living with unresolved stressors? Do you have neck tension that could restrict blood flow to the base of your brain, which is the area responsible for sleep regulation? (explained in an earlier section on concussion). If you answered yes to any of these, you might like to resolve them first, then check your sleep patterns again.

## INTUITIVE STRETCHING

There is a waking-up stretch that we all used to do every morning during childhood. It's the one children are pictured doing in storybooks. You know the one where you make fists, extend your arms way above your head, and yawn, stretching your arms skyward until you get that feel-good moment where the stretch takes over by going a little farther and then releasing. Then it's time for the legs. The curling toes and squeezing muscles get extended in the opposite direction until they can go no farther. You can even reach farther by stretching into your torso and side bending at the same time. This intuitive wake-up stretch that we all used to do every morning gave our body a total reset. Now we get so wound up, busy, and tired that we have collectively forgotten we ever did it. We stagger out of the bedroom and reach for the coffee instead. The other long-forgotten intuitive stretch is the one we used to do once standing after a long time sitting. You can help your body to remember this by standing with your feet slightly apart while rotating your hands outward with straight arms. (It helps to clench your fists.) Hold this pose while bending just a little backward. Amplify the intensity by taking and holding a breath while switching on all of the muscles you used to adopt this pose a little more. You will feel your automatic stretch response kick in. (Going up on your toes at the same time also helps.)

Animals stretch every time they begin to move after a long rest. Our cat is a stretch master. She begins with a very wide jaw-stretching

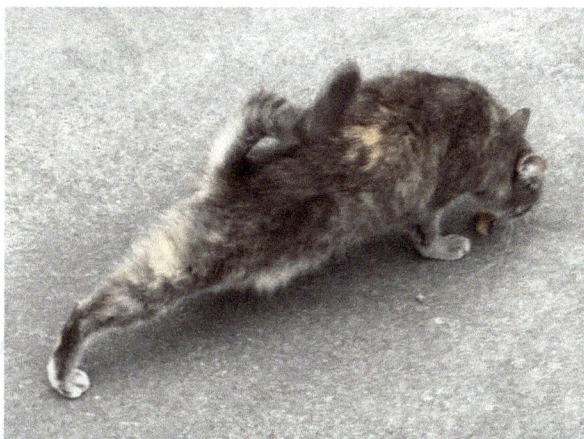

yawn, the perfect back-arching cat stretch, and then a downward dog. These are always followed up by a couple of individual back leg extensions. Only when fully stretched out does she walk off. She doesn't do this stretch routine every now and then; it happens every time she has slept for more than about an hour. It is an important part of her intuitive self-care routine and used to be a part of ours. This squeeze and release technique is not only great for our muscles; it also helps us to feel more positive.

Another day stiff, sore, and tired can transform into something that feels invigorating and refreshing. After you have done a few mornings manually, your automatic stretch response will take over. This will then happen every morning, I know it is challenging, but you have to remember to pause for a wee while and give it a chance to begin. I'm no sleep expert, but here are a few things that you can do to get that all-too-elusive good night's kip:

- Stop what you are doing about thirty minutes before you go to bed, particularly if you have been using a device or watching the TV.
- Dim the lights in your living space for half an hour before entering your bedroom. Use side lamps only (no overhead lighting).
- Play some relaxing, repetitive music (with the sound down low).

- Sleep stories or repetitive sound apps work for some people.
- Never look at the time if you wake through the night (timekeeping sets your body clock to wake at the same time the next night).
- Keep a notepad beside the bed and write down a bullet-point list of anything that is on your mind to be stored there for the next day.
- Go back to sleep using the controlled breathing technique, *counting to one* (see Chapter 19).

If your body pain is keeping you awake, it's a given that your posture is less than ideal. Following the simple suggestions in this next chapter will assist you in proper body functioning as well as sleeping soundly.

# CHAPTER 16

# POSTURING

## COMMON LANGUAGE

*"You're going to have to learn to stand up for yourself!"*
*"I'm just being up-front."*
*"She keeps me on my toes."*

## QUICK FIX

If you are out of whack, you cannot have fully functional posture. The foundational shift pulls you not only down but sideways as well. Stand, walk, and run slightly forward of center. Never pull your head in or your shoulders back. Raise your chest by being up-front, then, using devices, drop your chin toward your chest using the scull drop hinge only. Do daily planks to strengthen your core.

We don't think of our necks as being particularly powerful, and for a long time I wondered what sort of loading they could handle. Maybe they do need special support because they are fragile? That was until I took a trip to Bali. The containers in the image on the left are full of wet sand. These loads are somewhere between forty and fifty kilos (around 90 to 110 pounds), and I watched as it took two of them to get each one up high enough to be balanced on the head. Then off they would go! We came back around an hour or so later, and the whole pile, which was about ten cubic meters, had been shifted.

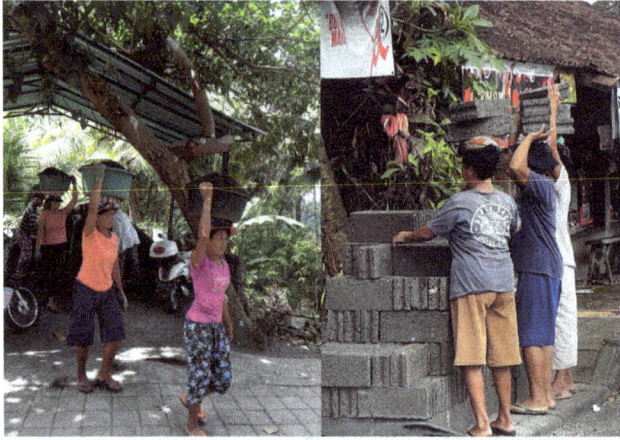

Later that same day, we came across women using the same technique to shift concrete blocks three at a time. The most astounding thing was that these were not one-offs. These women do this regularly. Take a closer look at the pics and you will notice their perfect posture and balance, which is the only way to do this work safely.

We used to crouch or stand with our torso forward, resting our knuckles on the ground. In this position our ribcage and shoulders were fully supported and our neck was extended in a continuation of our spine. Our head hinged forward at the top neck segment, allowing us to look ahead, opening the front of our neck.

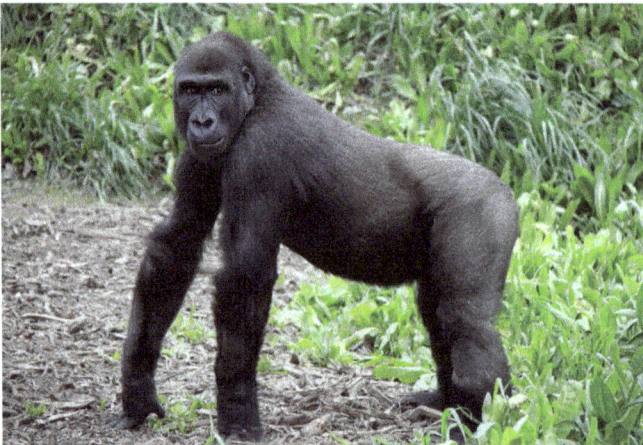

*Picture is courtesy of Orana Wildlife Park Christchurch New Zealand.*

As already mentioned in Chapter 3, somewhere along our evolutionary journey we decided to stand up. This enabled us to cover greater distances, getting around much faster with our torso balanced above our extended legs. But in doing so we lost support. Now we sit and stand with a collapsible abdominal gaping hole in the front of our skeletons. Remove the front legs off any chair and it drops forward and down, and that is exactly what happened to us. Our upper body, supported only by the spine at the back, dropped forward. This put a kink in the middle of our spine, squashing our abdominal contents. In doing so, it forced a compensatory backward kink in our necks. This neck overextension created a similar crushing effect, only in the opposite direction. Our shoulders, having lost ground support, responded to gravity by swinging forward and down.

*Rotate this next pic clockwise until the black line is horizontal. You will see that the model's neck is bent so far back already that returning the midsection of her neck to vertical has her actually looking toward the ceiling.*

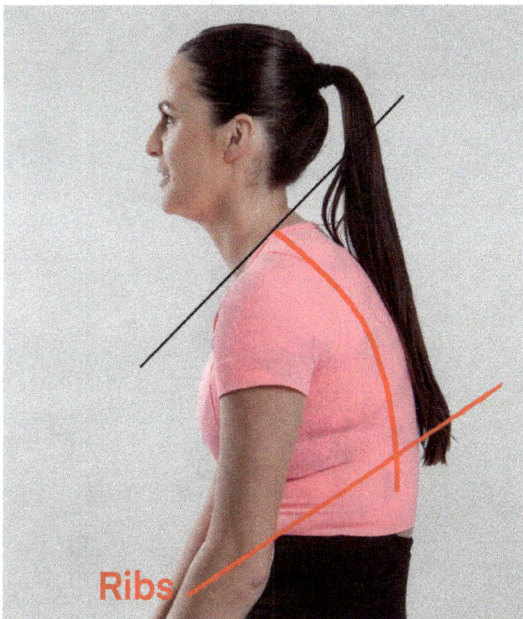

## BEING UP-FRONT

*Never pull your shoulders back or your head in! Get seated, then slump down into your worst posture with your head and shoulders forward and feel the strain the moment you try to pull your shoulders back or head in.*

This may have seemed like an obviously simple fix to those giving you well-meaning advice. Because your head and shoulders are forward-leaning, it makes sense to retract them, but this creates unnecessary tension in the upper back and harmfully further overextends your already extended neck. All you ever needed to do was lift the front of your ribcage.

*Now sit up as tall as you can and you will notice that your shoulders hang off the sides and your head sits on the top, no straining and minimal holding required. This perfect-posture silver bullet is what I have named "Being Up-front."*

*Locate the bottom of your sternum with your finger. It's at the bottom of the rib cage above the navel. Focusing on this point, raise it*

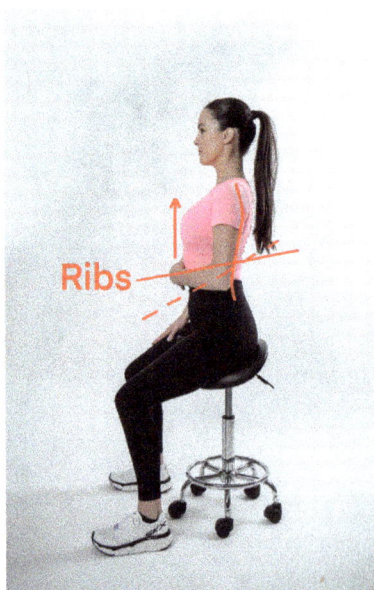

*upwards until it stops lifting. Take your hand away and sit in this upright position (just like pigeons do) for as long as you can. You will have to keep repeating this technique over and over, but as your postural muscles regain their natural strength, it will eventually become your new normal.*

## CORE STRENGTH

If ever there was a misleading slang term when referring to our bodies, it has to be *core strength*. You can never strengthen your core because you don't actually have any core muscles. Every time I went to a yoga class and the instructor started asking us to focus on our core, I had to bite my lip because, having studied our 200 bones and 600 muscles, I knew there were none there! To understand instructions, I have to be able to draw a picture in my mind. Apple cores are in the center of apples, and I knew that area in my body contained my stomach, intestines, bowel, bladder, and a few of my vital organs. *"Strengthen your barrel" would be a better description*, I thought. What we call our core is actually made up of sheets of very thin muscles crisscrossing the outer edge of the gap between the ribs and pelvis. This part cylinder is further supported by the abs at the front, and the spine and spinal erectors at the rear. The psoas muscles often bundled into the core description are actually our largest hip flexors.

*You may be able to feel some of your actual core muscles switching on and off by lying on your back with your fingers resting on your belly while slightly raising and dropping your head. Now roll over onto your tummy and try to hold a plank.*

If you can suspend your body between your outstretched hands and toes for three minutes tremble-free, you're strong enough. Any less and you have work to do. If you failed, you're normal. Most of us don't have a strong core, but don't fret. There is a very simple fix. Just keep doing planks.

## MARY

*"Planking has changed my life. I have been doing them every day for three weeks now, and my hips and back, which used to be sore all of the time, have stopped hurting!"*

It's really important to note that due to reciprocal inhibition, which I will explain later, your tight back can switch off your core. Any static tension held in your lower back switches the abdominal muscles off. That's why it is crucial to stretch and release your back when attempting to restore your weakened core. Another good reason to sit up instead of down is the crush on your lower back. As you slump down, sitting on your back instead of your butt, the pelvis rocks backward, relying on vertebral muscle strain for support. Short-term damages include lack of blood flow, compromised breathing, and abdominal congestion. However adopting this as your default posture will eventually cause disc failure and spinal bone deterioration. To have furniture that properly supports you while you sit, you need to know the difference between couches and slouches.

## COUCHES & SLOUCHES

Most of the furniture currently available is designed to look great in the home but is poorly engineered. The seats are too low and the backs are too far back.

There is a massive hole in the market for lounging furniture that actually supports us. What we really need are sofas and lounging chairs that are designed primarily for how they work rather than how they look. The base needs to be short enough for our bum to make it to the back support and high enough (without sagging) to hold the upper leg at least level. Even better if it's slightly downhill from the hip to the knee.

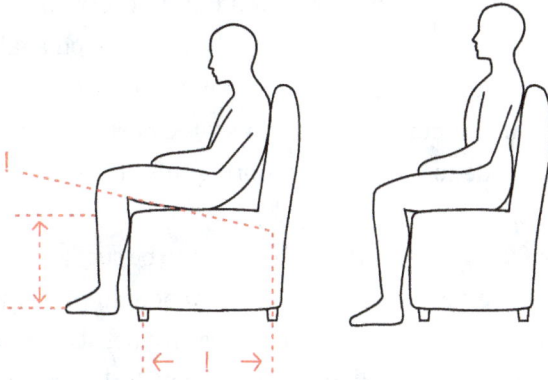

SLOUCH    COUCH

## SADDLE UP BAREBACK

I don't know if you have ever seen a chiropractic "sit right" chair. Available from about the mid-eighties, they were and still are brilliant! There is no back to lean on. The seat base is angled forward, slanting the upper leg downward, softening the lower back angle, and supporting the lower leg. The only downside was it being fixed rigidly facing

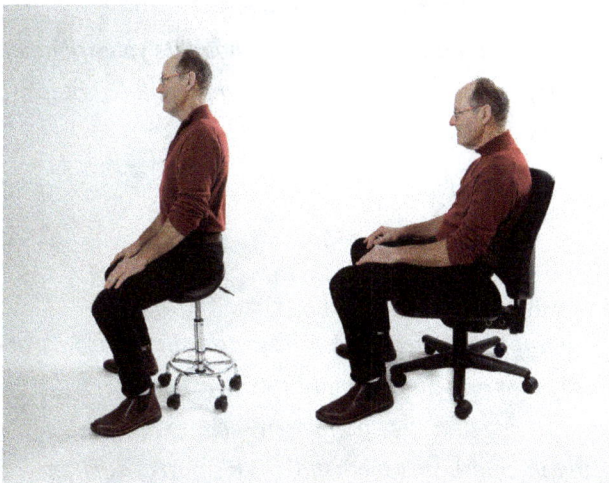

forward. You see, these chairs had rounded wooden blocks instead of wheels and no rotational ability. That's where the saddle stools came in. These chairs are revolutionary, and I think every able-bodied person should have at least one. With no back to slouch against, femur downhill to the knee, center rotational and wheels, they tick all of the boxes necessary for comfort and offer seated postural perfection. Our bodies were made to move, and adopting this active seating position achieves that.

In order for any postural improvement to be successfully adopted, there needs to be a corresponding improvement in your thinking. You must stop *bringing yourself down*. Repeating negative thoughts can encourage your posture to become *deflated*. This physical collapse, once adopted, can then prevent you from feeling and thinking positively. To counteract this, design a personal positive statement to pair with being up-front. It's a bit like mentally plugging a bike pump filled with self-esteem into the abdomen and giving it a few good pumps every day. As the muscles gain strength, so does the mind. After all, the mind does control the body.

## CONSTRUCT A VERBAL ANTIDOTE

*The first thing is to identify the negative thoughts you are having. Write any negative repetitive thoughts on paper, then build another statement in the opposite direction equally as long.*

### MARY

Negative (ailment)

*"I feel so unappreciated. It doesn't matter how hard I work or how much I do. My boss and the company always expect more. I've been doing extra work at home and they don't even seem to notice. It's time for my appraisal again, and I can't see it making a scrap of difference. Everyone else gets pay rises, but not me. My husband and kids are the same. They just sit around watching crap on TV and playing video games while I run*

*around doing everything for them. I'm sick to death of it all!"*

*Positive* (antidote)

*"I am so appreciated. The company and my boss are always impressed by my achievements and notice all of the extra work I am doing. I'm looking forward to my appraisal. It's their chance to let me know how well I have been performing. I won't be surprised by the offer of more money. Even though they seldom verbalize it, I know my husband and children appreciate everything I do for them. Taking care of them fills me with joy."*

Once you have compiled the antidote paragraph, it's a good idea to refine it down to a brief statement containing only its essence. It needs to be one sentence that can become a *verbal pill* to counteract negative thinking in the same way as sitting up opposes the slouch. This is difficult to do at first, but the most effective way is to look at your eyes in the mirror while reciting the statement out loud. Depending on your surroundings, this "pill" can also be taken silently.

"Everything I do is noticed, appreciated, rewarded, and feels really good."

*(Take twice daily with a glass of water.)*

## WHAT'S HOLDING YOU BACK?

As you defensively fold your arms, rigidly lock your knees, and "bend over backward," the entire static weight of your upper body is forced down onto your lower back. If you asked me how to ruin your back in the shortest time possible, I would suggest you stand like the woman in the image opposite. It would not be a case of "try a few of these and see how you go" because this will definitely do it!

By bending over backward instead of balancing, you force your hip flexors into locking on. Without them, you would fall over backward with your legs still upright (not pretty). Because the muscles holding you up are frozen in contraction, blood flow fails and they squeeze the life out of the lower back at the same time.

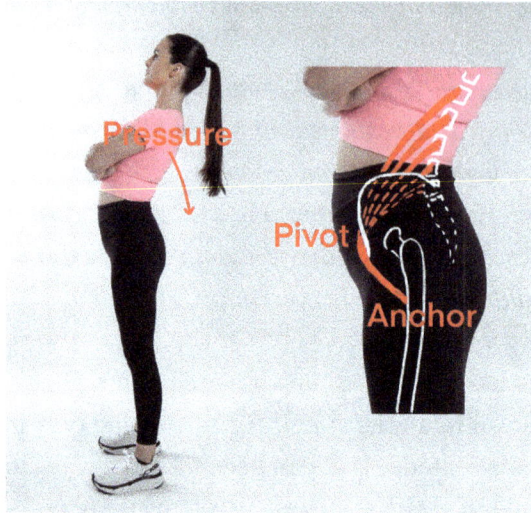

Grab a household broom and hold it at the end of the handle with the head up toward the ceiling. As long as the broom handle is vertical, it takes very little pressure to keep it there.

Now keep your hand where it is and allow the head of the broom to move off-center and you will feel instantly why you should never stand like this. The farther over the broom head gets, the harder it is to hold. In this scenario, your clenching fist represents your lower back. The way to

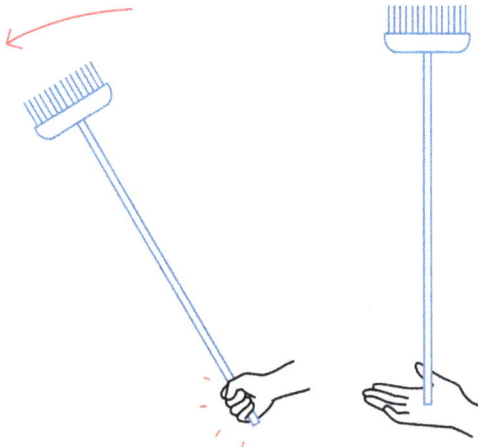

unlearn this destructive stance is to begin what I call standing upright.

## STAND UP-RIGHT

*Stand lightly to attention with your weight on your heels. Next, leaving your feet where they are, tilt your body forward until you almost fall over. Then come back just a little, stopping with your weight on the front of your feet but not the toes.*

Although this feels a little strange, it is the most functional position. Given time, you will get used to it. The next level is to walk forward while maintaining this same angle. It does take a lot of practice, and when you have this mastered, you will be ready to apply the same technique to running. I have found that people struggle for a while and usually give up, so in an attempt to make this more achievable, you can try to stop yourself from falling forward.

## STOP YOURSELF FROM FALLING FORWARD

Many people have a poor walking technique resulting in heel strike, and this simple technique totally alleviates the problem.

*Begin again by standing lightly to attention. Allow yourself to fall forward, thrusting your foot out in front of you at the last moment to stop yourself from actually falling. Then all you need to do is keep repeating this, one foot at a time, all the while, gradually increasing your speed.*

Walking or running, you will notice complete relaxation in your back. By lifting your chest a little at the same time, you will feel your abdominal muscles gently waking up as they switch on to become an integral part of your movements. Once engaged, your obliques provide

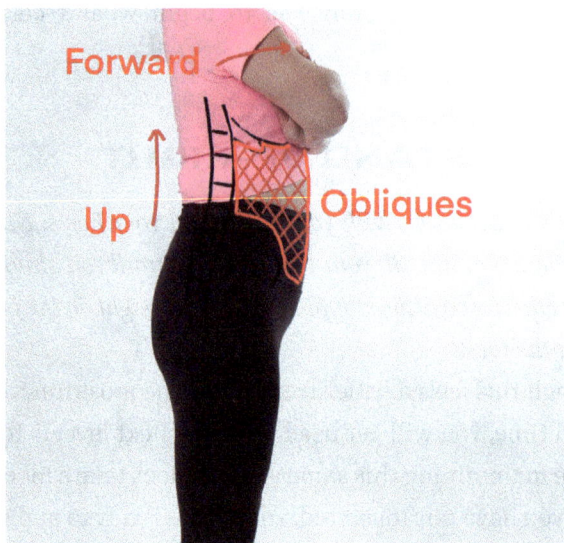

the half-barrel-shaped platform for the ribcage to rest on. This brings with it an enjoyable feeling of upper- to lower-body connection and relaxed coordination that has to be felt to be understood. As you stand, walk, and even run with your upper body weight actively supported forward of center, your lower back is actually being lengthened instead of crushed the whole time.

## DEVICE NECK SAFETY

With the current epidemic of upper-body pain and dysfunction caused by sitting with our heads down and forward, glued to our devices, we need a solution. With a steadily increasing supply of attractions to keep us drawn in, our devices see us hunched toward them more often and longer. One client told me that her daughter spends up to seven hours a day on five different platforms on any given weekend! Neck strain is happening the whole time our average five kilo head is suspended forward. You can avoid this by utilizing the top joint of your spine.

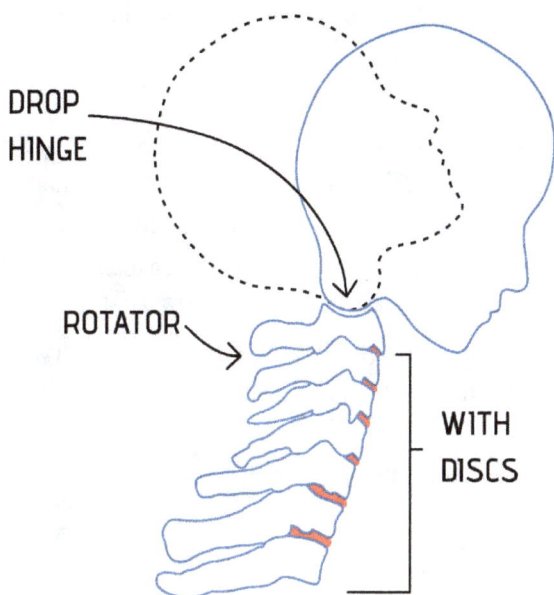

*To locate this joint, sit up and nod your head as far as you can up and down without moving your neck. The top joint that you have just located is the only one you need to use. The total solution is to be up-front first, or possibly even recline back a little, then look down by allowing your chin to fall toward your chest.*

## DOWAGER'S HUMP

This rather unsightly bulge is another cause and effect of the forward head posture. Our body is programmed to strengthen any area that is under impact or constant strain. Martial arts exponents know that if they hit solid objects repeatedly, they build a protective layer of scar tissue over the points of impact. This strengthening is not done to a plan; the body simply pours a few wheelbarrow loads of concrete into the affected area with the reinforcing rods chopped up into the mix. If your head is suspended forward for prolonged periods, this strengthening brew is applied at the base of your neck. The longer the head stays in that position, the more concrete gets poured in. Remedy this by sitting up-front and get a few deep-tissue massages to break up the concrete lump, and your body will clean up the residue (see Chapter 19 on "butterflies").

Although awkward at first and difficult to master, postural improvements are worth the effort, delivering balance instead of holding. Once established, your body will last a lot longer, trouble-free. Moving on now from external factors to the single-most important consideration for internal body comfort and longevity. You may be surprised to discover that this is *water*.

# CHAPTER 17

# WATER: THE DRIVING FORCE IN NATURE

– Leonardo daVinci.

## COMMON LANGUAGE

*"She's so brittle. Push her too far and she'll snap."*
*"He's such a dry bugger."*
*"Fluid movements."*

## QUICK FIX

Humans are made up of nearly 60 percent water. Without it, we are dust. Initiate your new water habit with a daily shot glass, taken morning and night.

Take a pic of your tongue and the inside of your mouth and you will see that it's all wet. We never think of what's inside us because we can't get a true view, but our insides need to stay as wet as our mouth, and the only thing that can do that is water. If the inside of your mouth dried out, you could not swallow and your tongue would snap off, and so it is for the whole rest of your body. It all needs water, not just to stay alive but to function. But this does not only apply to us, every living thing needs water. Not just most things but *everything!* Even plants living in the driest places on earth need water to live. Over their evolution, plants have come up with clever designs to catch and store even the minutest drops of dew that form on them in the desert. You will already know how important water is to your body if you have been for a long walk or a bike ride on a hot without any.

In the beginning, *the only liquid we used to drink and still need to this day was water.* In its purest form, water passes easily and quickly through our gut wall and into the bloodstream where it is transported all around. If it is anything but pure, it first needs to be filtered. The more we add to our water the harder it becomes for our bodies to access it. This internal filtering slows things down significantly. I'm sure we would get frustrated if we had to stand by a filter thirsty, with a glass at the bottom, watching the drips. Yet, thinking mostly of our eyes and taste buds, we have conjured up a ridiculous array of variations on the original theme of water, contaminating the original and slowing down its transition into our bodies. Next time you go to the supermarket, have a look at the number of different drinks. It's staggering what we have done to water in the name of sales and marketing.

*You may not want to go to the trouble of pouring an energy drink into a glass container and leaving it until the water has all evaporated, but I did just that. What you will see if you do this is that once the water has gone, the surface is coated with dye. It looks pretty on the shelf, but why would you drink that much coloring unless you wanted to change the color of your insides?*

## CONFUSION

On receiving a signal from our body, we chose how to respond, but it is possible for us to get it wrong. Feeling cold encourages us to put on extra layers. When we are hungry, we eat. When thirsty, we drink. But what if we get it wrong? I can remember decades ago, repeatedly going to the kitchen in search of something to satisfy what I thought was hunger. Nibbling on cracker biscuits and leftovers seemed to momentarily satisfy my desire, but why was it only temporary? I tried seeds and nuts, but still I was unsatisfied. Somewhere deep down inside me came the message, "I'm still hungry." One evening when feeling this "hunger," I drank a glass of water. Instantly, the craving stopped! I had been confusing thirst with hunger! So next time you're heading for the pantry, try the tap.

## HYDRATION VS. DEHYDRATION

Imagine for just a moment that you are a feijoa. A very strange suggestion, I know, especially if you have no idea what a feijoa is, but for the purpose of this exercise, just about any juicy, ripe fruit will do. The two following images are of the same piece of fruit before and after dehydration. This process removes enough water from the fruit for it to keep in a moisture-proof glass jar for several years as opposed to less than a week in its original fully hydrated state.

As I stated earlier, our bodies are nearly 60 percent water. Without water, we would be close to one-third of our present body mass!

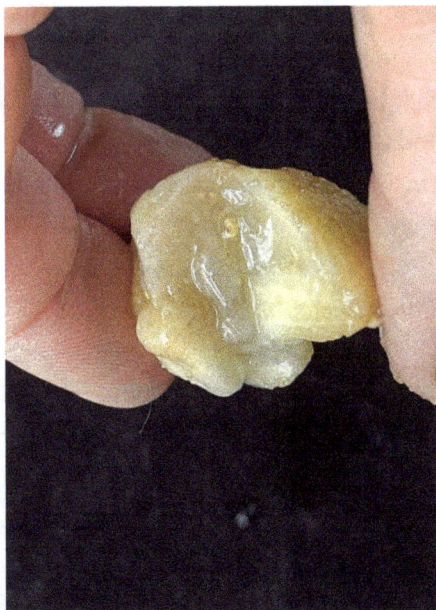

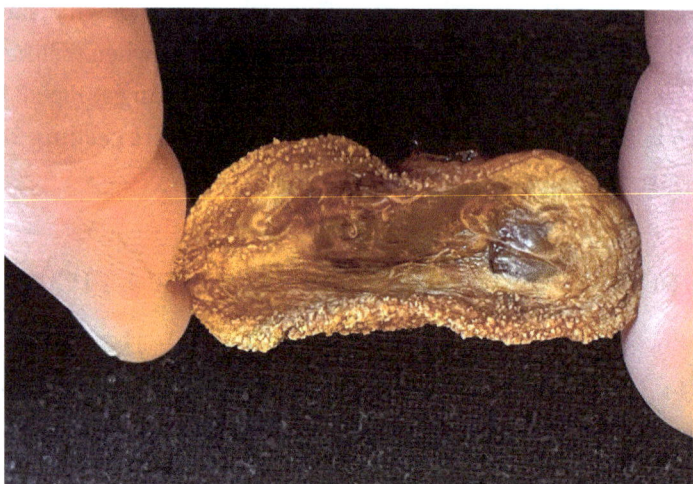

Looking up body facts, I was surprised to learn that even our bones, with all their rigidity, are one-third water. Getting back to the fruit . . . I could have used meat, but I know at least some people prefer not to be faced with the stuff we're made of. I chose these two images to represent just how important water is in our bodies. The fresh fruit is plump, soft, juicy, and easily pliable to the extent that it is difficult to grasp. Yet this same fruit, minus water, is the polar opposite. It's so hard that a firm squeeze on either end of the one pictured actually hurt my finger and thumb.

*This may sound like a silly exercise, but to gain the full experience you may wish to buy some dried fruit. It really doesn't matter what sort. Take it in your hands and get the feel of it. If properly dehydrated, it will feel hard, brittle, and fibrous, and require very little effort to break into smaller pieces. If you squeeze a sharp-ended piece between your finger and thumb, it may actually start to generate pain.*

*Now drop it into a bowl of water and leave it to soak overnight. Then drain the fruit pieces through a sieve and hold them again in your hands. When gently pressed and released, they will have a natural tendency to submit to the pressure and bounce back to their original shape, undamaged.*

Our bodies are not fruit but are nonetheless made up of organic material that responds in a very similar, if not the same way to hydration and dehydration. If you were either one of these pieces of fruit, what would life be like as the dried one? With a dehydrated body, movement in any direction would be difficult, painful, and cause internal wear and tear. Without water our brain cannot function. Remove the liquid or gel from any battery and its output drops to zero! Therefore, in order to have this organic computer of ours working to full capacity, it is essential that it is properly hydrated.

*Just like in the experiment with the dried fruit, a glass of water taken before sleep will effectively soak our brain overnight so that when we wake the next morning, it will be fully hydrated, plump, and completely functional (potentially anyway).* This makes it less likely for you to stare into the distance, chewing your pencil, with your thoughts lost along a dusty highway.

Now before you say, "I can't do that because I'll be up all night peeing," there is a way. Of course, if you were to go from nothing to drinking a large glass of water before bed, there is every chance of you being up at some ungodly hour having to empty your bladder. Start small. Because our bodies, given the chance, are relatively quick to adapt, start with a shot glass and build up slowly from there. The amount matters a lot less than the timing. Do this every night, and you will soon start to feel like the shot glass is too small. Once this happens, you're off into a new, healthy habit. By increasing the amount a little bit at a time, your bladder will adjust with you. Another of water's important functions is cleaning.

Imagine for just a moment being filthy on the inside. We have all heard of the importance of fiber in the diet. It's a bit like eating a scrubbing brush. But unless you add water, all the scrubbing does is move the dirt around. Have you ever had a shower without turning on the water? While doing the dishes, the first thing we do is fill the sink with water. Maybe a little too much information here, but flushing the toilet is probably the best analogy when demonstrating the importance of water for internal body cleansing. You can push the button as many times as you like, but without water in the system, nothing moves. This is exactly how it works for your body! The next time you have a shower and come out all clean and fresh, you might like to drink a glass of water to wash your insides as well. Kidneys filter the blood, but what cleans the kidneys? The short answer is water. Urine is mostly water and can do no cleaning and waste elimination without it, and I think at this stage you will agree that hydrated number twos move a lot easier. So if you have time to read the paper before you're done, maybe add some extra $H_2O$ to help move things along.

## WHAT ABOUT THE BLOOD?

If you were to tip a jar of honey upside down with the lid off, it would stay in the jar for a while. But if you stirred in even a small amount of water, you would increase its viscosity, which helps the honey to flow. Add a lot more water and you could easily tip it from one jar to another. You have probably all seen your own blood on the surface of a minor cut, which comes out dripping and quickly sets. There are platelets in the blood designed specifically to block any holes in the system, like cuts, scrapes, and the like. The rest of the setting is just the blood drying out. Without the water, it becomes almost solid. Drinking less water thickens your blood, making it harder for your heart to pump the blood around. The larger vessels close to your heart offer very little resistance to blood flow. But as it travels farther away, just like the branches of trees, those vessels carrying the blood get smaller and smaller. The tiniest of these are called capillaries, and there are bazillions of them. Every part of your body needs blood to survive, and these minute pipes make sure it gets to and away from the cells living in even the most remote extremities of your body. Any viscosity reduction places strain on the system and slows everything down, and at the very least would cause fatigue. The most extreme example of this flow restriction is frostbite, where tissue actually dies. If the pipes were all open and the blood was thin enough to flow easily, the extremities would be maintained at the same temperature as the body's core because blood distributes body heat.

## H₂O BEAUTY THERAPY

I wonder if any of these skin-hydrating beauty products actually hydrate the skin. Maybe rub some on a piece of dried fruit and see if it softens. I think the answer is quite simple. If you take another look at the fruit, dried and hydrated, the surface tells the story. Hydration comes from within. Beef jerky is meat with the water removed. If you bent a piece of dried meat forward and back even a couple of times, it would probably snap. Dry skin becomes hardened and wrinkly, just like dried beef, but drinking even a small amount of water daily might be enough to keep away those fine lines that appear on the "before" ads for skin-hydrating beauty products. This water, added through the bloodstream, hydrates the emerging new cells rather than wetting the dead ones on the outside that are about to fall off. The surface layer of our skin is dying and shedding at the rate of about 35,000 cells every minute. That adds up to about four kilograms every year of dead skin that has fallen off of you. (Apparently, this dead skin is responsible for most of the dust in our homes.)

## LIPS

I don't know if you suffer from dry, cracking lips, but if you do, it can be very uncomfortable. In the worst cases, they can even split open. There are plenty of products designed to combat this lip drying, but I never use them. I see my drying lips as an alarm to let me know that I'm either stressing out or running low on H₂O. Stage fright causes dry mouth and lips, but dry lips from working outside on a hot day can be remedied by drinking a glass or two of water. Some people's lips will dry out faster than others, but the same basic principles apply to us

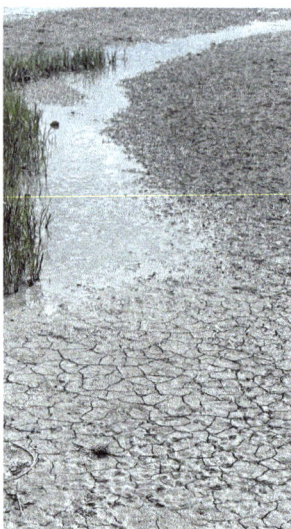

all. This pic is taken at the edge of a lagoon where the tide is receding. It's taken on a fairly hot day, and what was soft, fine mud, the type that could easily squish between your toes, has gone hard and cracked. These cracks did not happen slowly over time; the water had only just receded! The soft, squishy mud hasn't gone away; all that is missing is the water. These cracks have formed as the surface dehydrates and shrinks, just like the cracks that form on our lips and skin.

## HEADACHES & BREATH

On a summer's day after running around outside and bouncing on the trampoline, my stepsons would more often than not come to me complaining of a headache. My answer would be, "Try drinking a glass of water, and let me know if your headache doesn't go away." The next time I would see them would be hours later when they had come in for dinner. They hadn't felt thirsty, but all of that exercise on a hot day used up enough water for their head to let them know they were running low. Every time this happened, a glass of water was enough to make the headaches mysteriously disappear. As we breathe during exercise, we expel water at the rate of about 60 to 70 milliliters per hour. I don't know if you've ever been skiing or snowboarding, but the water vapor leaving the body while we breathe is easiest to see when the outside air is really cold. Condensing as it cools, leaving our warm interior, it looks like we are breathing out fog or mist. We need to replace the water we breathe out and, because we breathe a lot more while exercising, our need for rehydration is increased.

Drinking more water will effectively rehydrate all of your muscles, right? Wrong. Compacted tissue cannot be better hydrated just by drinking more water. The static tension held in those areas very effectively excludes any extra water we drink.

*Fill the kitchen sink with water and dip in your clenched fist. Then remove your fist and open it up.*

The water has not gotten in. Even though your fist was totally submerged, it is still bone-dry on the inside. That's what it's like for our compacted muscles and joints. It does not matter how much extra water we drink; if the area is too tight, water fails to get in. You could pop your clenched fist into the ocean and, even though it is submerged under the largest visible body of water on Earth, it remains dry on the inside. The only way to let the water into your hand is to release the tension and let it open while still below the surface. And so it is for muscular and joint tension. The only way to hydrate a compacted

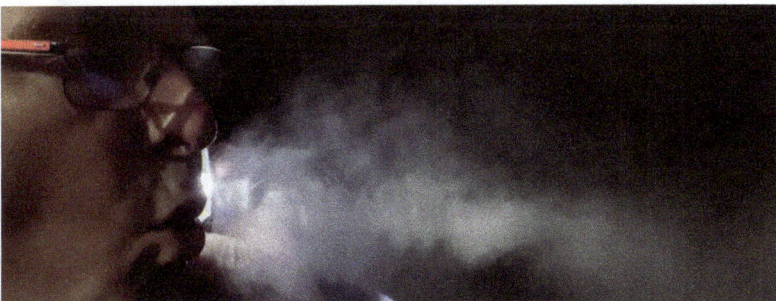

muscle is to release the tension that is keeping the water out. Before leaving this subject, let me add a quick note about why *dehydrated muscles can snap*. It usually happens seemingly without cause. You could be jogging along, low on water, and hear/feel a pop in your upper leg as a muscle ruptures completely. The muscle I'm talking about, one of the quads, sits in the middle of your upper leg on top of the other three quads running from the front of the pelvis to the top of the knee and is usually a bit dehydrated and tender already. Having a tendency to be one of the most compacted muscles in our body makes it a dehydration injury risk.

*Sit with your knee bent to 90 degrees, run your thumb across the top of your thigh, and you will feel this quad. Instead of being soft and pain-free, it is probably tender to the touch and feels firm, more like the handle of a small baseball bat.*

Right! I'm off to drink a glass of water and then write about food.

# CHAPTER 18

# FOOD FOR THOUGHT

## COMMON LANGUAGE

*"I can't eat that. It doesn't agree with me."*
*"I'm so glad you're safely home.*
*My stomach was tied up in knots."*
*"Forgive me I am having a little trouble*
*digesting what you are saying."*

## QUICK FIX

Refined foods burn rapidly, exploding inside us, initiating and accelerating inflammatory diseases. Consume a balance of slow foods (foods that release energy gradually) eaten slowly in moderation. Then you can stop spending so much money (116,000,000 NZD annually) on supplements that are mostly available in whole foods.

Electric cars have the plug on the end of the wire so that the wires can't get mixed up. This setup also stops people from getting electrocuted. But the most important reason for the design is to prevent people from plugging it into the wrong power supply, which could blow the car's electronic brain or set it on fire. It's a similar scenario for a petrol or diesel vehicle. If we load in the wrong fuel, either the engine won't start at all, or may even over rev and blow up. Unfortunately for us, that's exactly what we are able to do with the food and beverages we consume. We don't have a food-specific aperture. What we do have is a taste-sensitive, saliva-metering grinder at the entrance to a chute. This is why we are able to consistently get it wrong with food. You don't have to be a nutritional expert; it's been drummed into us over and over. Fresh fruit, vegetables, protein, and water should be the key staples in our diet. What you may find useful is to pause long enough to determine whether the food you are about to consume will fuel or foul you.

## THE LUXURY OF FOOD OBSESSION

You decide every day what your trillions of body cell residents get to eat. For the most part, they are at your mercy. Sure, they do occasionally throw it back up the chute if it's contaminated or pass it on through as fast as they can. But the rest is up to you. They can't make you into a silk purse if you feed them a sow's ear. I call food obsession a luxury because our ancestors were forced to eat produce that was able to be grown or sourced locally and in season. In *Rachel Hunter's* Television New Zealand Series, *"Tour of Beauty,"* she interviewed some residents of Middle African civilizations that are still fueled by little more than dates, milk, and goat meat.[1] These she describes as some of the healthiest-looking people she has ever seen. The Eskimo people lived well on mostly meat, fat, and seaweed. Their summer diet extended to include grasses, berries, and some plants. Back in the day, if you chose not to eat what was available locally, you would die of starvation. To make seasonal foods last longer, they were either dried, salted, or coated in fat. But now, thanks to transport networks, processing, and refrigeration, food is everywhere you look. We are relentlessly bombarded with foods, fads, choices, trends, and diets. Micro packaging of individual portions that each create their own landfill. Modified, refined, stripped, and chemically enhanced, we are confronted by an ever-expanding list of unhealthy options. Our local supermarket now has fifty-six shelves of sweets and sixty shelves of potato crisps. The owners of some food-processing businesses and corporations, driven solely by profit, are tempting us through our taste buds and our eyes, all the while costing us more for less food value. Peter says that with some of these foods, you are probably going to get more nutritional value by throwing away the contents and eating the cardboard box. I will stay away from any temptation to mention brands here, but the latest trend is making the packaging much bigger than the contents. The stand-out here has to be biscuits (or cookies to some) that are held on a forty-five-degree angle to maximize space, hiding the fact that there are only six in each packet.

Then there are shrinking containers. Cans that used to be 500, 200, and 100 grams are now 425, 185, and 95 grams. Another popular way to rip us off is to increase the ratio of advertised products to water. For example, canned tomatoes actually listed on the label as being only 60 percent tomatoes! Then there are the canned beans which can be as low as 40 percent beans. Toilet paper and paper towels are not embossed to help you. The embossing means that the manufacturer can use less paper. Look at the end of any roll of embossed paper and you will see the gaps in between the layers. While you are looking at the end of the roll check out the hole in the middle. Yes it

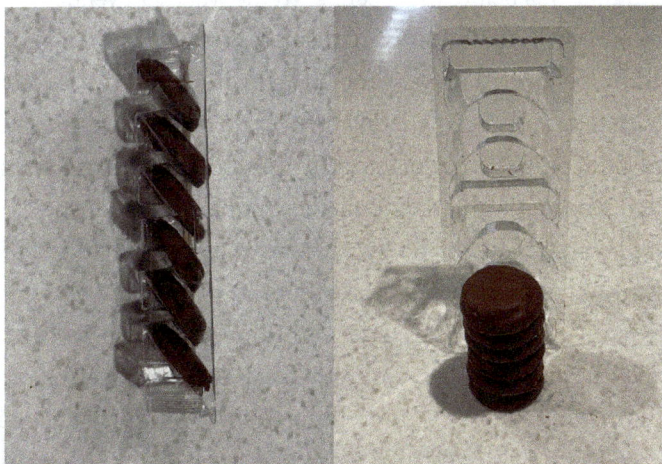

has been made bigger! None of this is done by invaders from outer space; we do this to ourselves. The people controlling these organizations are human and entirely responsible for the multitude of ever-expanding choices available to us. Apart from farmers markets, they collectively design, manufacture, and control our consumables.

If you want to get an idea of how big and bad they can get, have a squiz at *Grapes of Wrath*, a book by John Steinbeck. It's a very frank account of what was actually happening with food control during the Great Depression in America in the early twenties. It tells of corporations piling fruits and vegetables into mountains and pouring kerosene over them. Slaughtered animals were dumped by the truckload into shotgun-guarded rivers. All this was done in an effort to keep the price of food high when people were starving to death.[2] Hugh Fernley-Whittingstall and Jamie Oliver have both done courageous TV exposes taking the current corporate model head-on. The very real difficulty that we face as consumers is the ridiculously high price of healthy, whole foods. Currently in New Zealand, we are having our wallets squeezed by two supermarket giants. Their duopoly gives them an unfair advantage, which is now public knowledge, and they seem to have adopted a "screw them while you still can" attitude. One example is what seemed like too highly priced cauliflowers at $4.00 each, which went up to $8.00 the following year, and that was before the recent extreme weather events.

Country of origin is another consideration when purchasing food. Thankfully, chemicals used by the farmers of Aotearoa, New Zealand, are regulated, and those chemicals proven to be most harmful are banned altogether. In an attempt to protect consumers from food imported from unregulated countries, mandatory country-of-origin labeling was introduced. Sadly, there is a thing called "made from locally grown and imported ingredients," which effectively sidesteps the whole purpose of the regulation. Why should we be concerned about food imported from unregulated countries? Because substances proven to be harmful to humans may have been used in the production. Simon Reeves, intrepid explorer and documentary maker, stumbled across a caviar farm in a Russian lake that was warm in spite of snow right up to its shores. He discovered that the lake was being heated by the outflow from a nuclear power plant which was rapidly described as *safe* by his guide.

A lot of what is currently happening with food is actually our fault. We get the final say by what we buy or choose to leave in the stores. We consumers actually control the industry. But the food choices that were driven by our bodies' needs have shifted into our heads. Just like our breathing, it all got lost upstairs. Our senses of taste, vision, texture, and smell, which used to help us discern whether food was in a fit condition to consume, are now driven by desire. How it looks, smells, tastes, and feels in our mouths is now driven by our pleasure centers. We have collectively lost sight of the fact that food is meant to keep us alive, maintain our bodies, and fuel our movements. Why food for thought? Because your brain accounts for a mere 2 percent of your body weight but consumes twenty percent of your calorie intake.[3] By consuming foods with little or no actual goodness, your brain will fade. In our natural world, we harvested meat, nuts, fruits, and plants. These were consumed very close to their original state and were probably just called *foods*. These originals are what we now call *whole foods*.

Jim Blair, a ninety-two-year-old masters games athlete, was featured in our local newspaper in 2024. He looked to have a physical age of about sixty-five and believed in keeping things simple. In what he called common sense, he suggested avoiding diets, fad or not. "I just eat normal food, whatever is available," Jim said. "Being less active in winter, I put on a bit of weight, but that falls off in summer when I do more."

## WHOLE FOODS

Take a close look at some of the more common nuts and seeds. Tough on the outside, soft, fibrous, and oily on the inside. They are alive. Unprocessed and given the right conditions, they will grow. These little gems contain nutrients that are released slowly. They first have to be ground between your teeth, and, when mixed with saliva, any food value held in their fibrous bodies is gradually liberated as they travel through the digestive system. If you were to chew on raw sugar cane, which is a bit like soft bamboo, you could slowly get the sugar out, but it takes an awful lot of gnashing, and the fibers have to be spat out. Refined sugar, what my father called "the white death," can be swallowed without chewing and explodes inside you like a Molotov cocktail. *Boom!* You get all of the energy at once and then it's gone. This explosion plays havoc with your body and mind. Highly refined foods burn us from the inside. Inflammatory diseases appear or flare up once sufficiently fueled. This also applies to alcohol, which, if lit, will actually support a flame. Sugar is cheap, delicious, and fun to eat. I don't know if you've ever picked up children after they have been to their grandparents' house, or tried to settle them after an evening of trick-or-treating, but chances are they will be on a sugar high. Like a blowfly on a string, they buzz around and around until the sugar runs out, eventually crashing off the other end of the high. This is what it does to our insides. Trillions of cells buzzing around out of their tiny wee nuts, then crashing, waiting for the next hit. Yes, sugar is a drug, and now you have to go and find some more because, like all drugs, this one is highly addictive. It's not just sugar; these same principles apply to any foods where the energy has been stripped from its slow-burning original container (white flour).

The graph opposite shows two lines, both representing the release of energy from food. The blue line is for unrefined foods. Because the energy releases slowly, there is no spike and it never enters the higher output red zone. The black line representing highly refined foods changes to red as it spikes in a fast-release phase before crashing and stopping short.

The answer for the cells in your body and for children is the same. To stop them from rushing around like mad things and then crashing, give them whole foods.

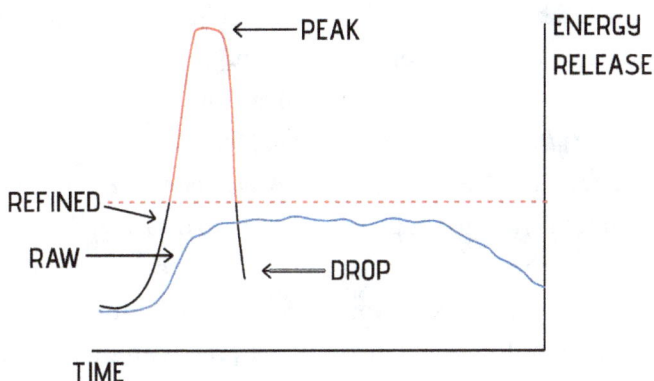

## JUICE

Put any food through the juicer and you're probably better off eating the contents of the bucket on the side. What you have just done is separate the slow from the burn and make yet another form of rocket fuel. The solution? Eat whole fruit and vegetables. Our local school could join the revolution here by renaming Fruju Friday to Fruit Friday.

## OBESITY

Our body fat is potential energy. For 200,000 years we struggled to feed ourselves, and we needed fat to keep us alive when food was unavailable. This hard-wired us to accumulate calories. We are perpetually surrounded by food now, and therefore need to override that programming. A quick glance at our body's fuel gauge (our beltline) tells us whether or not we have enough in the tank. If it's running low, we need to eat. Any junk in the trunk and we need to move more. It's really not more complicated than that. Yes, I realize with the rapidly spreading problem of obesity that I've just poked a stick into a hornet's nest. But the fact is, if you leave a petrol engine running and don't refill the tank, it will eventually run out of fuel, and so will we. If you don't believe me, check out the reality series *Alone*.[4] Contestants are dropped off individually into the freezing wilderness and eat only what they can forage and hunt. One by one, they are uplifted after failing health checks, mainly as a result of malnutrition.[5] Diets don't tend to work for long, but there is a very subtle change that can help.

*Each time the desire to eat something unhealthy or more than you need strikes, take a five-minute pause.* Because our age-old habit surfaces on impulse, a pause is usually enough to disarm it. If you decide after that time that it's still going down the chute, then so be it. But a lot of the time the pause will work. This moment in time gives you the opportunity to shift the idea from your tiny reptilian survival brain to your big brain where it can be rationalized.

## PRESERVATIVES

A simple test for the preservative level in any food is how long it will last at room temperature. The longer it lasts the more chance of it containing potentially harmful substances. Several items of takeaway food have become infamous for lasting years and even decades unrefrigerated. Thanks to refrigeration, we no longer need to eat chemically processed meat, but we still do it because it has so much flavor. Pickles is another one. Back in the day, pickling was a valuable tool used to extend the shelf life of perishable foods, but now it's mostly fun for our taste buds.

## STRESS

What we are thinking at mealtime matters so much more than what we eat. There are countless diets out there, promising to be the one to make you thin and healthy: total carb, zero carb, total deep-fry, zero nightshades, pro-dairy, dairy-free, vegan, vegetarian, carnivore, keto, fasting, zero sugar, zero fat, eat fat, pescatarian, wheatgrass. I hear even zero water is now a thing. But no matter what eating style or fad diet you choose, if you are not in a relaxed state when you eat, the food is mostly wasted. As already mentioned in the fight-or-flight chapter, stress and fear shut down digestion. Maybe there's a hole in the market for pre-digested food. You may laugh out loud, but who knows; it could soon be another fad. Then busy, stressed-out people could squirt a tube of it down the hatch and keep rushing around, knowing that their body could still soak up some goodness.

## IDEAL DINING

*Turn off the TV, the video game, the phone (actually turn it off), and come back to the dining table and focus on eating your meal. Then, once a week eat a fully nutritious meal. All of your body cells will celebrate for its goodness. From there, increase it to twice a week, and continue to build on this until your diet consists of mainly high-quality meals.*

## NEXT-LEVEL DINING

*A fun exercise to help let go of your stress and reconnect with your food is to prepare a meal that presents no burn or spill risk and then eat the whole thing with your fingers, eyes closed. To gain the most from this experience, choose some food that needs to be chewed. Attempt to keep your mind aligned with the textures and tastes of every mouthful.*

The sheer number of exercises and stretches in Chapter 19 could easily be overwhelming. Just pick one or two to integrate into your day and add others later on.

# REPAIRS AND MAINTENANCE

## COMMON LANGUAGE

*"Use it or lose it."*
*"I need to bring myself back down to Earth."*
*"A stitch in time saves nine."*

## QUICK FIX

Incrementally get good at what's good for you. To integrate improvements, choose one or two activities from this chapter to do every weekday for two months. Once you have achieved that, add another one or two.

Your body and mind are inseparable. A frozen mind freezes the body, and a body, once frozen, shackles the mind. Freeing one releases the other. This chapter on repairs and maintenance contains a series of micro improvements. Avoid the boot camp approach to mind- and body-enhancing improvements. Too much done too soon creates more pressure on our already pressured existence. The following list is specifically designed to be *gradually* integrated. You can drastically improve your overall health very simply by incrementally integrating these tiny positive adjustments into each day. You may not be able to find the time to attend a weekly yoga, pilates, tai chi, or stretch class, but you can take a ten-second breath to look over your shoulder almost anytime.

## ERADICATION THROUGH HONESTY

Do what you've always done, and you'll get what you've always got. It is important to work out how you got stiff and sore. We can be oblivious to our own negative traits that are glaringly obvious to those around us. Find the inner strength to admit to yourself that you are not perfect. Then you can find and weed out the things that hinder you, systematically replacing them with functional habits.

## COMFORT

In order for your body to relax and let go, you need to be comfortable. A number of the activities listed in this chapter will involve you lying down. Floors are hard and tend to amplify already painful spots, so you may have to use some form of padding. A yoga mat may be all that you need, but if your pain level is really high, you might like to use a self-inflating roll-up tramping mattress. If you can no longer make it down onto the floor, do some exercises while lying flat on your bed.

## SAFETY

Never push any movement into pain. If you feel that any of the activities offered in this section are causing your level of discomfort to increase, *stop immediately.* Often you will discover that moving in one direction is pain-free and the other is not. Because it's not possible to move one side of the torso in isolation, any body movement in the pain-free direction helps to free the other side anyway.

# REPETITION

Repetition entrenches behaviors, both good and bad. It makes no difference whether things help or hinder us; anything we do a lot of gets easier to repeat. We choose whether we get better at rushing, chilling, panicking, cruising, forcing, easing, obsessing, trusting, overeating, fasting, and rationalizing ad-infinitum. When asked, "How many times do you want me to do my stretches?" I usually answer, "Some." Most clients who tell me that their physiotherapist couldn't help them admit to having done their all-important homework a couple of times and then stopped. Generally speaking, those who do their homework daily are the ones who get better. It's also a good idea to take weekends off. It helps to have a break and a fresh start. To avoid falling off the wagon, think about how many times you could incorporate positive tweaks into your worst day. Then set a little less than that as your starting point. Your successes will fuel your progress. Do not increase your baseline target for two months. After the eight weeks, increase your target but only to what you can achieve on your worst day.

## PETER

*"You are amazing! I have been everywhere and tried everything, but for the first time in as long as I can remember, I am getting better." In his mid-sixties, Peter was chronically restricted. His steadily decreasing physical ability was slowly but steadily shutting him down. Having given up on ever playing golf again, his walk was reducing down to little more than a shuffle. After the first few sessions and being "very skeptical," he admitted to feeling a little better. This switched on the possibility of recovery, and he locked into doing his homework every day. He bounded through the clinic door on his twentieth appointment, ecstatic about*

*what amazing abilities I had. "I have just shot a ninety at golf, and it's all because of you!" Highly motivated by feeling improvements, Peter had done his stretching and exercising many times every day and was reaping the benefits. Sure, I did assist his recovery, but had he not done the bulk of it himself, I would probably have been added to his long list of practitioners who had not been able to help.*

## GETTING UNSTUCK

With a fear-filled life and a rigid body to match, you may think straight away that the only way out is to change your thinking, but there is another way through. Your body can actually help your mind to move on by reaching a little past where it was holding. With each subtle unfurling of your inner hedgehog, your mind, sensing the improvement, relaxes. All animals, including humans, have a built-in rapid-muscle release mechanism. None of the animals in nature have read self-help books on the best way to eliminate tension from their bodies; they intuitively utilize it, and so can we. It's simple:

- Gently access your perceived end of range.
- Breathe in, then hold and resist for ten seconds.

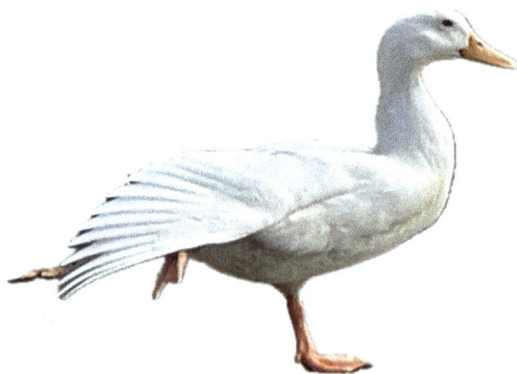

- Breathe out, following the release.
- Repeat three times.

1. **Gently access your end of range.**

   *Place your right hand flat against your right cheek, rotating your head left until it stops, and gently hold it there. Take a mental note of how far you can see to the left.*

2. **Breathe in, hold, and resist for ten seconds.**

   *Inhale fully while turning your head ever so slightly toward your hand, then hold for ten seconds.*

3. **Breathe out and follow the release.**

   *Turn your head left while breathing out, using slight hand pressure to rotate and hold your head a little farther left.*

4. **Repeat three times.**

   *Once is good, twice is great, and three times is complete.* Why three times? Even on the third cycle, the magic continues. Your whole body is wired to release by removing resistance. By choosing not to push into each stretch, the pushback is eliminated. All you ever need to do is invite the muscle to extend farther along its natural range. I have grouped together a set of release poses, all of which incorporate this technique, which I will now refer to as GBB3.

## LEG OVERS

*Lying on your back, hold a dumbbell or kettlebell heavy enough to hold your right arm down at forty-five degrees to the side of your neck. Use your left hand to bring your right leg over the body with your knee bent, encouraging it toward the floor. Apply GBB3. Repeat for the other side.*

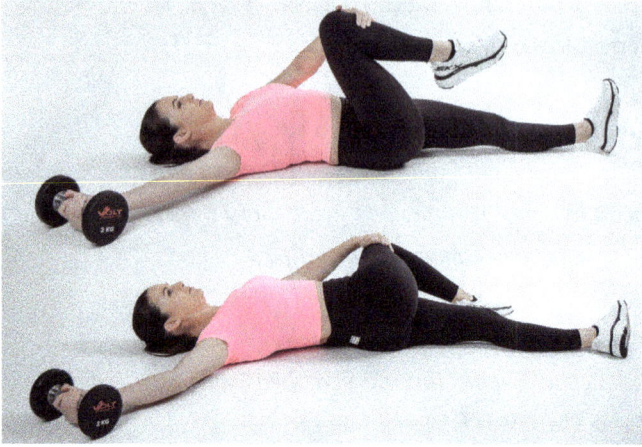

### Next Level

*By bringing the held knee closer to your head, you can move the release farther into the muscles around the hip. Extending it farther away shifts the focus up closer to your torso.*

## JUST PULLING YOUR LEG

*Lie down on your back and hold a bent leg just below the knee with both hands, fingers locked together. Apply GBB3.*

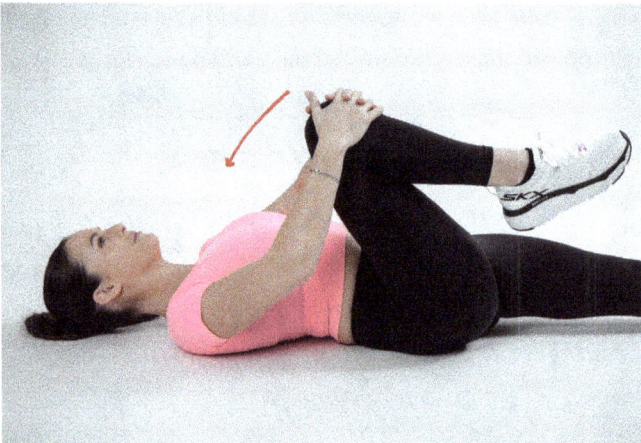

### Next Level

Once you have completed the third GBB3 cycle, lightly jerk your knee three times toward your shoulder to mobilize your SI joint.

# BUTTERFLY
## (device-related fatigue reset)

*Seated or lying down, raise your chest while locking your fingers together behind your head, elbows apart. Take a big breath in and pretend that you are cracking a walnut between your shoulder blades by extending both elbows as far back as you can. Push your head back into your hands and hold your chin up, then keep it there for ten seconds. Keeping your chest up, breathe out, bringing your head forward and down, closing your elbows together like the wings of a butterfly. Do three complete reps, allowing your upper body to follow your head forward on the last one.*

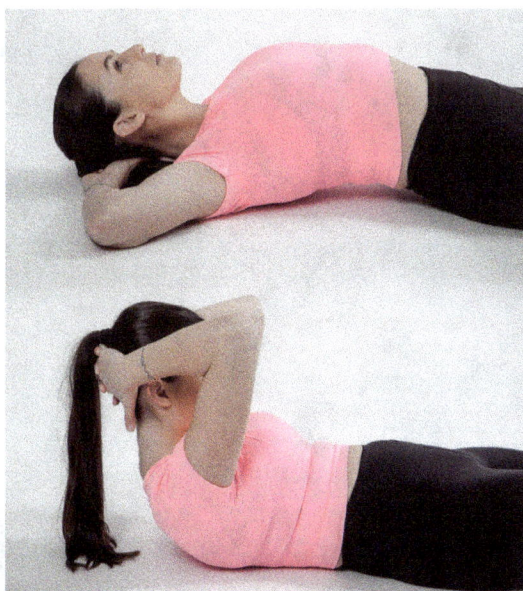

### Next Level

Begin the compression cycle with your head lightly rotated to the left. Apply GBB3 rotating further down to the left with each release phase. Repeat for right rotation. *By keeping your body upright while continuing the stretch, you can generate a very pleasant headache-relieving muscle burn. This you can learn to position into the sweet spot under the base of your skull or bending slightly forward, move the burn farther down your neck as required.*

# BEING UP-FRONT
## (perfect-posture silver bullet)

*Sitting or standing, place your index finger at the base of your sternum (bottom of your ribcage in the middle-front) and raise this point skyward. Push your chest against your fingertip, taking it a centimeter forward. Drop your hand and stay up in this position until you forget, then repeat.*

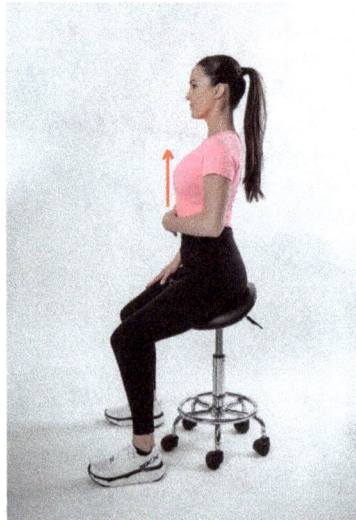

## SITTING DOWN
## (moving from your head into your body)

*Sit in a comfortable chair with both feet on the floor, hands separate from each other, eyes and mouth closed, focusing on your breathing. (Your breathing does not need to change, but it will probably deepen and slow down by itself.) You decide how long and how often to do this. To get started, begin with just a few minutes at the same time every day.*

## TURN THAT FROWN UPSIDE DOWN
## (Your body can be happy
## even if you are not.)

*Lie down, eyes closed, and smile while tuning into what is happening inside. You will feel the smile received by your body as you soften wherever you have been holding. Don't be surprised if you intuitively sigh.*

### Next Level

## THE OTHER PDA
## (public displays of acceptance)

*Learn to wear your smile publicly. This will feel a bit clunky and counter-intuitive at first, but very quickly it melts into a sumptuous, warm feeling that can be self-administered anywhere, anytime, even in the face of adversity. Smiling is like a magic trick. Your internal relaxation can be further enhanced by uttering a very gentle hum.*

## THE ATTITUDE OF GRATITUDE

*Choose positive thoughts. Are you a glass-half-full person, or do you see life through rose-tinted glasses? Call it what you like, but choosing to reframe your thinking is difficult to initiate. Just like physical exercise, though, the more you do the easier it gets. Even the tiniest positive thought proves that you can do it.*

## WASHING MACHINES
## (mobilizing your rusty hinges)

*Stand with your feet more than hip-width apart. Arms loose by your sides with toes turned slightly in. Turn your head, followed by your body, to look as far around as you can. Repeat in the opposite direction. Continue turning alternate directions while gently increasing the speed until your arms flail.*

## SACRAL SHIFTERS
## (groin pain and prostate)

*Stand with your feet hip-width apart and place both of your thumb tips side by side, pressing against the top of your gluteal cleft (builders' butt crack). Keeping steady forward thumb pressure, pulse your hips forward*

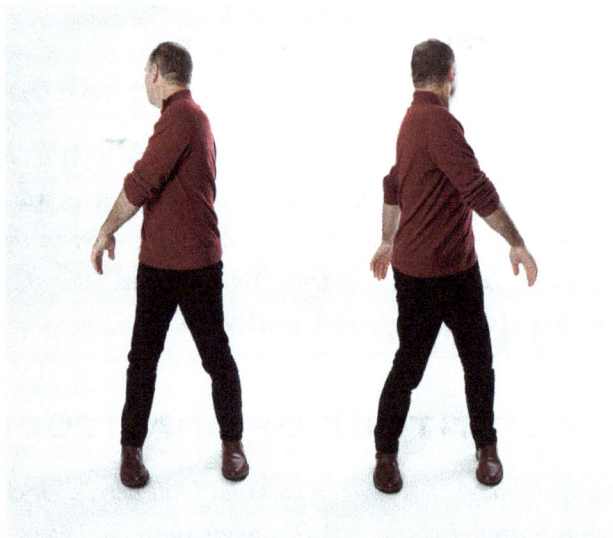

*and back 100 to 200 times. It's easier to count every second pulse. Near the end of the cycle, you will feel the hold of your lower spine soften, and walking will become easier.*

## THE SINK (sacral extension)

*Stand directly in front of your kitchen sink. Place your feet facing forward, a little farther apart than directly under your hips. Holding the front edge of the sink with both hands, shuffle your feet backward until your body is leaning slightly forward. Drop gently into a squat without lifting your heels off the floor and with your head down.*

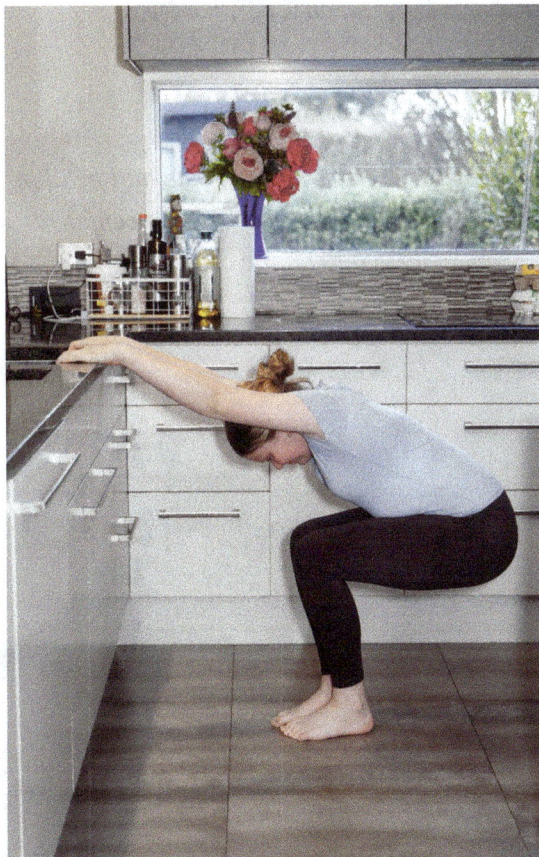

### Next Level

*In ten-second cycles, breathe deeply into the stretch, allowing your body to rise following the in-breath, then fall with each exhalation. Shuffle your feet slightly farther back and repeat.*

## FOOTY KICK
## (lower-back instant reset)

*Stand on one leg with the other extended behind you. Next, pretend to kick the ball over the goalpost. Then swing your left leg back to its resting place where it started. Repeat on your other leg.*

### Next Level

*Slowly at first, move your outstretched arms and head in the opposite direction as your leg swings forward. Once confident, increase the intensity while doing three reps on each side.*

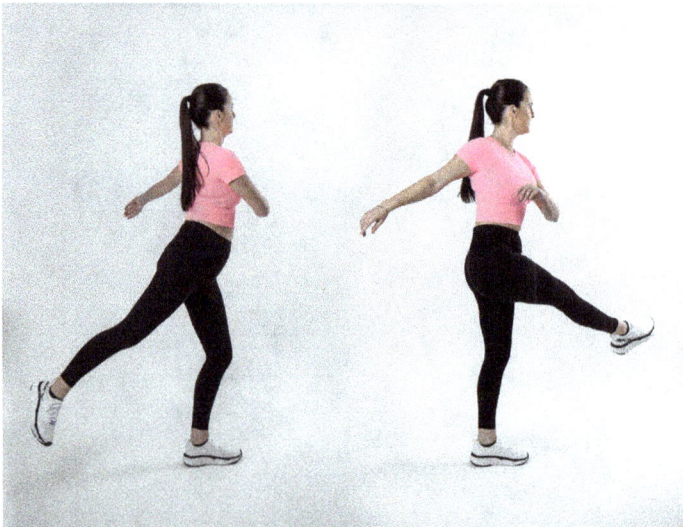

# LOOKING FOR SPIDERS
## (daily neck rotations)

*Every time you sit on the toilet, sit upright and look behind you as far as you comfortably can. After pausing for ten seconds, look around the other way and hold for another ten. Remembering in the early stages can be an obstacle, so pop a removable reminder sticker on the wall.*

*Tip: Another removable sticker on the wall behind you will help to track improvements.*

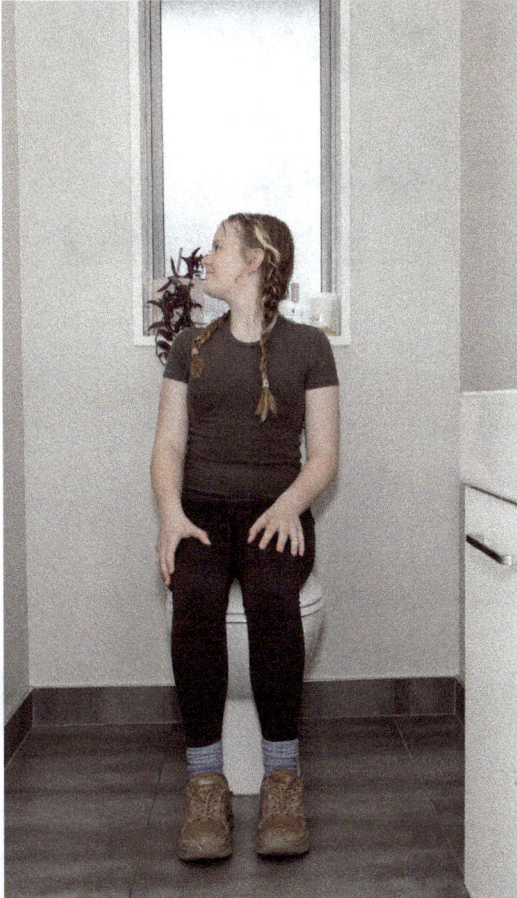

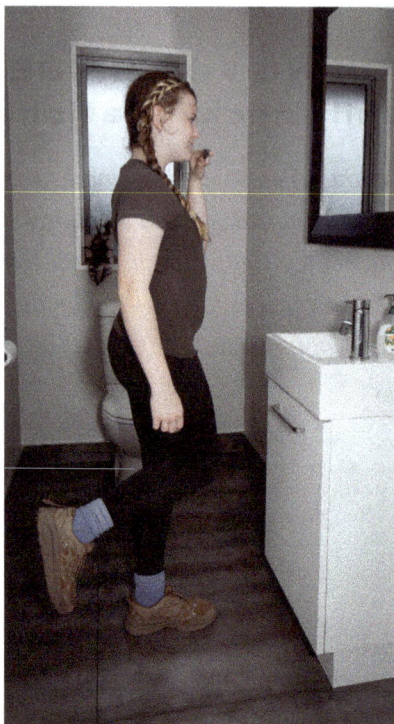

## STORKING

*Stand on one leg while brushing your teeth. Hop from side to side until you can stand on one leg for the duration.*

### Next Level

*Once proficient, either close your eyes or do one-legged squats while still brushing your teeth.*

## JACKHAMMERS
## (rapid reenergizers)

*Standing up straight as relaxed as you can, go up ever so slightly onto your toes and then, gently at first, drop onto your heels. This will send a wee jolt*

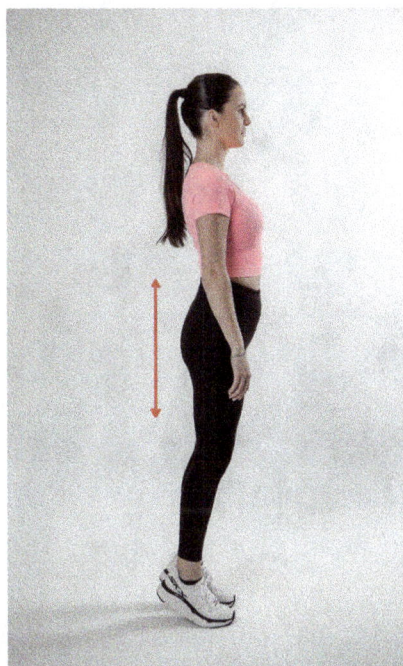

*to the top of your head and all the way out to your fingertips. If this feels okay and pain free, keep going, gradually increasing the rate and intensity.*

### Next Level

*Once proficient, increase the energy a little on the upward phase, lifting your feet just off the floor on each up stroke, simultaneously raising and dropping your arms like you are flicking water off of your fingertips.*

## YOU'RE SO VEIN
## (unlock lower-leg varicosing)

*Lie your upper body across a table with your legs spread, feet on the floor. Slowly creep your feet farther apart until you feel stretching on the insides of both legs. Hold for at least two minutes. Creep your feet back together before standing up.*

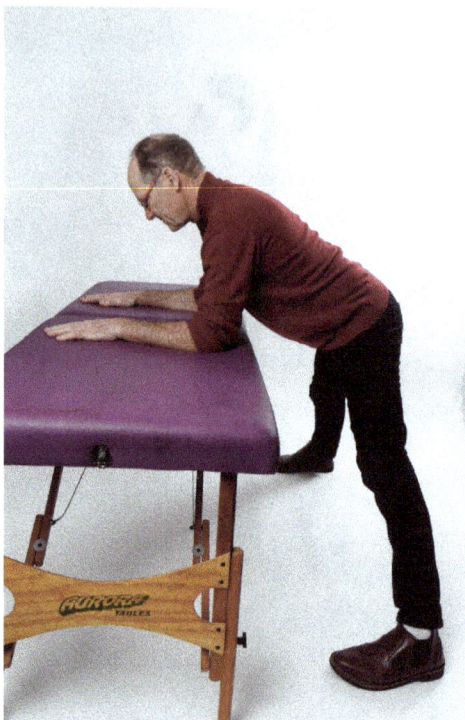

## TWO TOWEL RESETS

Never change the order of these movements!

   *1. Place a rolled-up towel behind your neck, holding the free ends in both hands.*

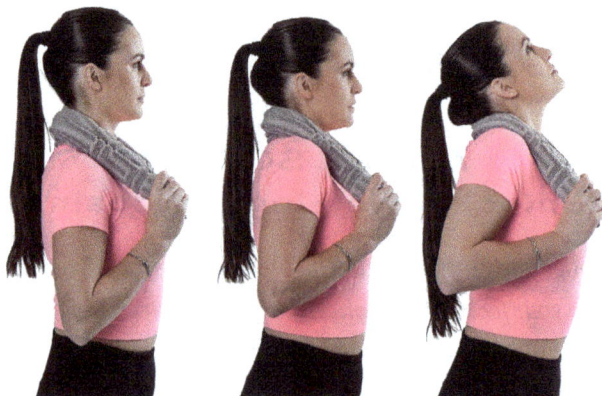

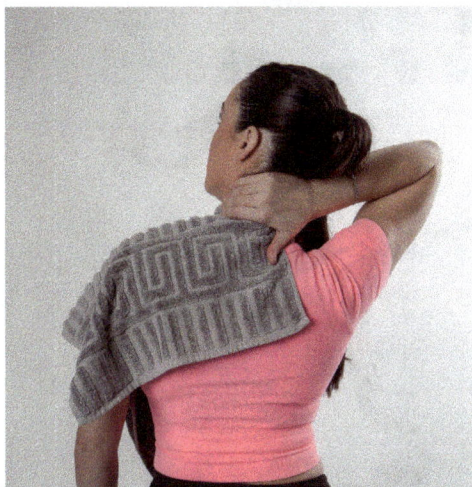

2. *Raise both of your shoulders up and back.*
3. *Once, and only when your shoulders are raised, tilt your head back and squeeze the towel between the tops of your shoulders and the back of your head.*

### Next Level

*After microwaving a much smaller dampened towel, roll it up inside your large towel and repeat the exercise. These neck resets are great preventative maintenance and also serve as a remedy for headaches and eye, ear, nose, and throat irritations.*

## THE OTHER TOWEL RESET

*Post shower, place the towel (single layer) on the left side of your neck, then reach over the top with the right hand and place your fingers around the neck with your thumb pointing down the spine. Clasp the whole area with your hand and pull forward and down. As your elbow moves toward the floor, simultaneously drop your head forward while rotating to look over your left shoulder. Repeat for the right side.*

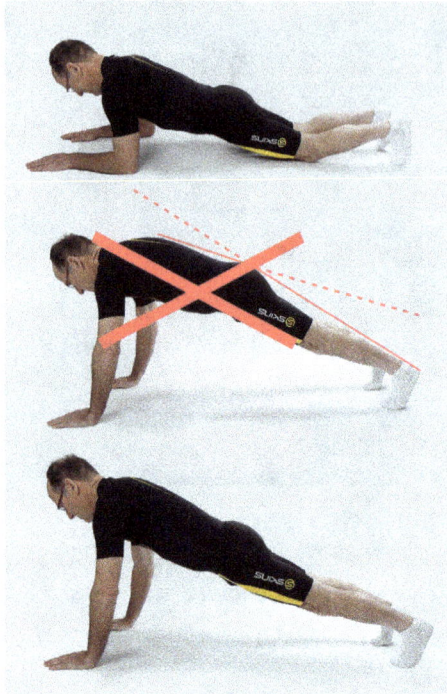

## Next Level

*Reach your free arm down and across behind your back to amplify the stretch.*

# PLANKS

*Lying flat on the floor, start with your elbows directly under your shoulders and raise your body up to a straight line suspended between your forearms and knees. Then lay flat to rest. If this feels easily manageable, extend the lift onto your toes, straight arms, and palms. Do three reps until you feel a tremble each time, resting flat on the floor in between. Use a side mirror or ask someone else to check that your back is in a straight line. The image in the middle is demonstrating how not to do planks. This upward bend is cheating by taking the pressure off a weak core.*

Next Level

*Keeping your legs straight, raise one foot, then change to the other. Once proficient, raise the diagonally opposite hand simultaneously.*

## WAKING UP YOUR WAKE-UP STRETCH

*To re-initiate your long-forgotten intuitive stretch response, breathe in, raising your hands above your head while pushing your feet as far away as you can. Then activate as many muscles in your back as you can recruit while bending slightly sideway.*

## COUNT TO ONE

This tool effectively shuts down stinky thinking, getting you to sleep or back to sleep. Do the counting silently in your mind.

*Breathe in . . . and . . . Breathe out. One . . .*
*Breathe in . . . and . . . Breathe out. One . . .*
*Breathe in . . . and . . . Breathe out. One . . .*
*Repeat until . . . ZZZZZzzzzzzzzzzzzzzzzzzzzz*

## COUNTING TO THREE

*Whether it's starting the car, answering the phone, sending a text, tapping your credit card, talking, or you are engaged in any action except hitting the brakes, stop what you are doing and count to three.*

### Next Level

*Next time you think that you are really busy, try stopping what you are doing and count to sixty. This is really hard to do. Did you get angry? Probably. Keep going. The calm is always there, waiting to be savored.*

## "ME" APPOINTMENTS & SAYING NO

*Put some gaps in every week labeled "me." Then, when any one of the approximately eight billion of us asks you to do something, you can honestly answer, "No, I'm sorry, but I can't do that. I would love to, but I already have an appointment. Is there another day or time that may suit?"*

## KEEP YOUR HEAD WHERE YOUR HANDS ARE

*Whatever you are doing (preparing a meal, pedaling your bike, showering, or even breathing) be there fully, feeling it all.*

## TUMMY BALLOONS

*In bed morning and night, lie flat and place your hand on your tummy. With your mouth closed, breath slowly toward your hand and let go twenty times.*

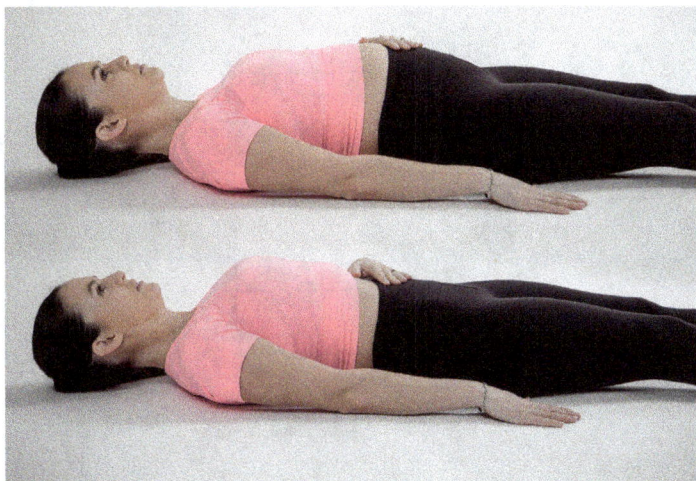

## ENDLESS IN-BREATH

*Gradually restore your entire breathing capacity by continually breathing in without stopping or holding. Count while you do this, repeating to at least the same total each time. Return to a normal breathing pattern with three rapid outward huffs.*

## STOP N DROP

*Endlessly breathe in while keeping your head where your hands are and you will feel your mind stop as you drop from your head back into your body.*

## GET OFF YOUR HEELS

*This very simple technique lengthens your back instead of crushing it. Standing upright, bring your weight onto your heels and then forward onto the balls of your feet (the large pad at the front behind your toes). Utilize this slightly forward stance whether standing, walking, or running.*

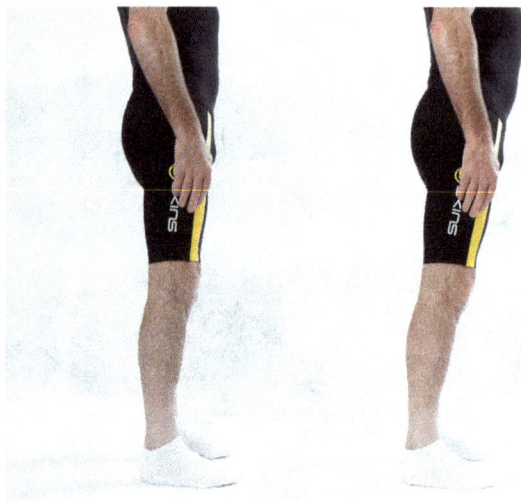

*There is an easy way to adopt this slight forward stance while walking. All you need is a day pack containing half a dozen full 1.5-liter water bottles on your back. The nine or so kilos will be enough to tilt the upper body forward of center, bringing the foot down flat onto the ground in front.*

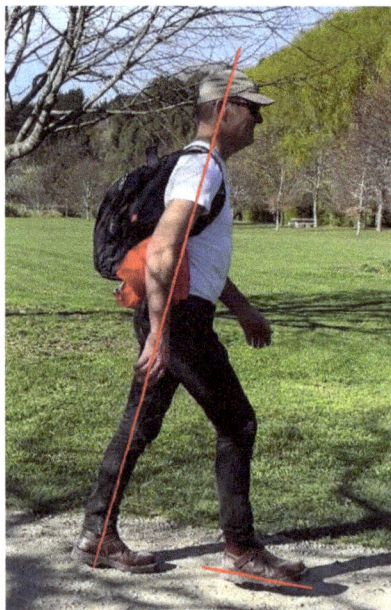

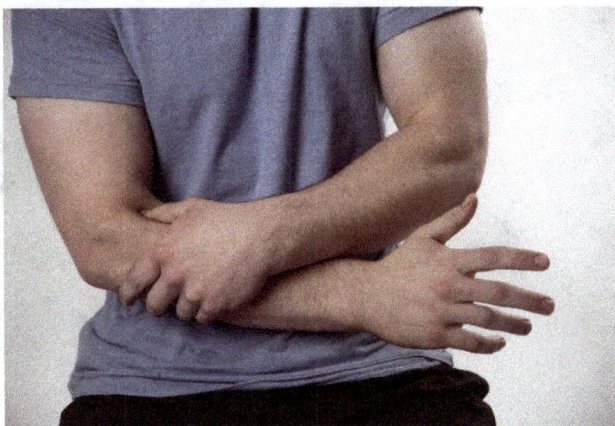

## TRAP AND WIGGLE
## (release compacted tissues and knots)

*Locate the most tender point on any muscle and apply pressure to it using your thumb, gently increasing the pressure until the pain elevates to a "good hurt" level. Open and close the joint past your thumb-pressured point until the pain drops to about half of what you started with. An example of this would be to trap a pressure point on your forearm and move your hand back and forth, bending at the wrist.*

## HAVING A BALL

There are all manner of fancy gadgets available to manually ease your body pain and suffering; some are very effective, and some are not. These next two self-treatments utilize a very simple and cheap tool available from sports shops: a cricket (or lacrosse) ball. Most of the dull pains felt in the front of your shoulders are actually being referred forward from pressure points on the muscles of the shoulder blade. You will also find that most leg pains can be relieved by releasing the tension you hold in the muscles above your actual hip joints. (As we stand with our hands on our hips we are holding the top of our pelvic bones, not the actual hips, see Chapter 1 for details.)

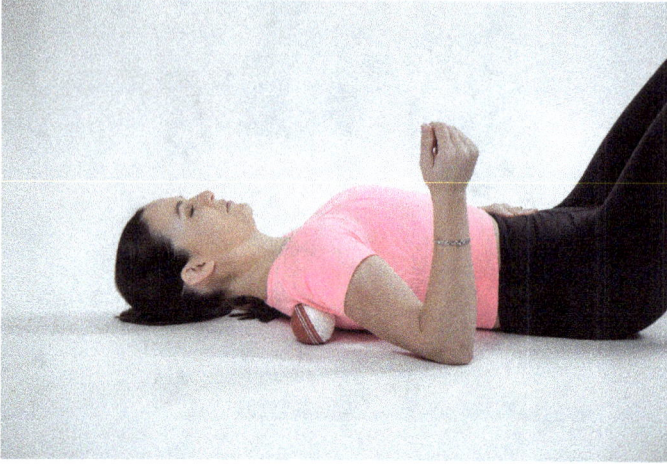

Place the cricket ball on the most painful pressure point on the shoulder blade, then, resting your elbow on the floor, move your hand back and forth to rotate your upper arm. Continue until the pain has reduced by 50 percent. Move the cricket ball to the most painful pressure point on your glutes, then keep your foot on the floor, move the knee of the same side left and right until the pain dissipates by about 50 percent. You may find up to three different pressure points in this area on each side, all referring to discomfort in your leg.

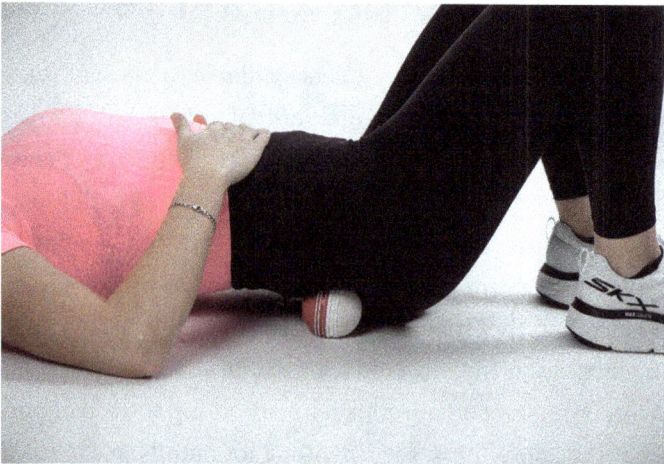

## ON A ROLL

The end goal here is to roll your back through its full length by lying on a foam roller, hands behind your head. It is a great way to treat compacted muscles in your back, and you may even release the occasional locked spinal joints.

*Begin by rolling the upper back and shoulders with your arms folded across your chest. Once this can be done pain-free, extend the treatment by moving the roller in stages farther down your back with each repetition. Once you can do this exercise from top to bottom comfortably, increase the effect by locking your hands together behind your head.*

### Next Level

*Try and touch the ceiling with both hands at once while rolling your upper back. Then position the roller at 45 degrees to your spine and repeat, to roll the muscles between your spine and shoulder blades.*

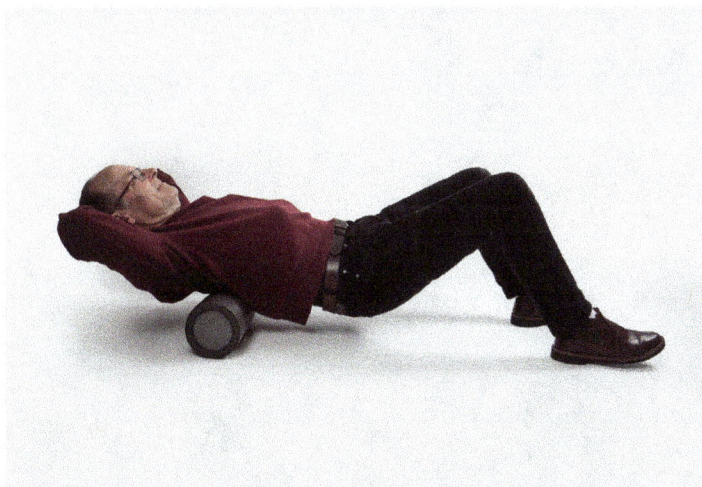

## THE ELIXIR OF LIFE

*Drink a shot glass of water at the beginning, middle, and end of every day. Do this in the same way as you would take a pill. Once this has developed into a regular habit, gradually increase the size of the glass. This health-enhancing habit can also be used to silence hunger pangs.*

Chapter 20 is all about the cause of our common colds. Like all good mysteries, once solved, the cause will seem obvious.

# THE CAUSE OF OUR COMMON COLDS

## COMMON LANGUAGE

*"You're really starting to get up my nose."*
*"Brace yourself against the cold."*
*"You're so irritating."*

## QUICK FIX

Stress, anxiety, bracing, and lower temperatures increase neck pressure point activity. The pressure points respond by radiating inflammatory referrals to the ears, eyes, nose, head, and throat. These remotely located inflammatory responses compromise pro-bacterial populations. This leaves the way open for invading pathogenic bacteria to proliferate. The best cough, cold, and drippy nose prevention is to eradicate pressure point activity and associated inflammatory referrals by regularly maintaining total neck mobility.

There's an old story about a drunkard who was looking for his lost wallet under a street lamp across the road from where he dropped it because the light was better. Up until now, the search for the cause of our common colds has overlooked his logic. The symptom-focused medical model has been searching in the most obvious place: inside our noses and throats. The problem with this search is its total focus on the complaint but never the actual cause.

There is a constant battle for supremacy going on in our throats and nasal passages. Apparently, we have billions of friendly bacteria of about 700 different types guarding this warm, hydrated bacterial breeding ground. With all of this localized protection, you might wonder how this defense system could ever be breached, allowing us to catch a cold. But it does and we do, in huge numbers every winter! All it takes to weaken our army of defense is an environmental shift. There have been volumes written about the location and treatment of the "knotty bits" in our muscles with their associated referral zones. Dr. David G. Simons, scientist, along with President John F. Kennedy's personal physician and medical researcher, Janet G. Travell MD, pioneered musculoskeletal medicine. Internationally recognized for their work mapping trigger points and referral zones in the human body, they co-published *The Trigger Point Manual* in 1994. Their trigger point manuals were an essential part of the teaching material used at the therapeutic massage college where I obtained my diploma. Their trigger point and referral zone wall charts are used internationally as a valuable visual reference in musculoskeletal and therapeutic massage clinical treatment rooms. My viewing of the cause of our common colds was greatly enhanced by standing on the shoulders of these two medical research giants. My personal preference is to call trigger points pressure points because our life pressures ramp them up, and localized mechanical pressure further activates and can be used to resolve them. They are the ruffians, the bullies of our bodies, and just like the bullies in our society, being compromised and weak, they become a painful irritation, radiating destruction to make their presence felt. There are lots of these in muscles all around your body, but the ones that cause headaches, itchy eyes, runny noses, swollen neck glands, ringing ears, and inflamed coughing throats all reside in your neck.

*To feel an example of this mechanism in action, gently yet firmly dig your thumb into one of your headache referral points at the base of your skull (bottom of the two images). Most of our headaches are generated here, and the one you may be able to feel, radiates up the back of your head, over your ear, and usually intensifies in the temple. Ease the pressure enough to slide your thumb directly forward until it comes to rest against the back of your jaw bone with the top edge still under your skull. This is the location of one of your throat-irritating pressure points, which will make you cough when you push and hold it.*

The throat and nasal environments need to be stable enough to sustain a thriving community of friendly microbes with populations dense enough to prevent infestation by colonizing invaders. It's the same scenario in our throats as for the gut bacteria. The analogy I used when talking about lack of gut health, where orangutans can't survive on a palm oil plantation that used to be their jungle, can also be applied here. Once the respiratory environment has been compromised, the survival rate of our pro-bacterial residents reduces, and the battle is lost. Referred inflammation from compacted neck

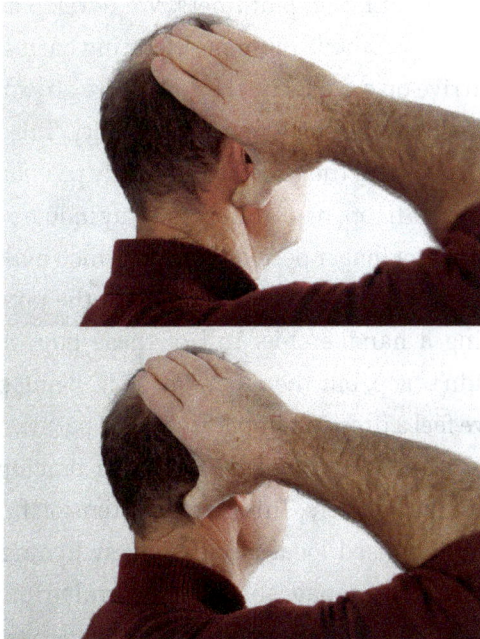

muscles inflames the respiratory passages, destroying the local environment. This leaves no more chance of the friendly microbes surviving than a koala after an Australian bushfire.

Those of us who are lucky enough to have been born into an existence totally below the red line can wander through fields of pollen-saturated grass without so much as a sneeze and will rarely if ever catch a cold. The rest of us who visit or live entirely above the red line are sneezing and coughing with red eyes and runny noses at the slightest provocation. So now, thanks largely to our steadily rising life pressures and habitual medicinal dependencies, neck tensions are allowed to ramp up, increasing pressure point activity. This causes remote referral sites to become increasingly inflamed. Because of this debilitating stimulus from these remotely located renegades, the throat and nasal-passage lining can become red and raw. This renders the unfortunate bearer hyperreactive to a few specs of dust. If this inflammatory surface disturbance is of sufficient magnitude and is persistent enough, the local environment alters to a degree where the friendly bacterial population plummets. We develop a cold once the critical threshold is reached. These proliferating harmful bacteria do not suddenly arrive on a cold day; they are there already in comparatively small numbers, waiting for an opportunity. This breakdown of our natural defense is all they need to suddenly proliferate.

So why does this happen in winter? We stay indoors a lot more and are closer together for longer periods of time, which makes it easier for germs to move from person to person. Before the popularization of tissues, carrying a handkerchief full of these bugs around in our pocket sure didn't help, but there is more to it. Being cold makes us tense. When we feel a drop in temperature, our natural response is to *brace ourselves against the cold*. It's this winter bracing that tips the scales in favor of the invaders. This increased tension further restricts the already-compromised local circulation, switching the pressure points from what was a manageable, mild referral to fully on. Whether it's individually, head, ears, eyes, nose, throat, or all together, whatever

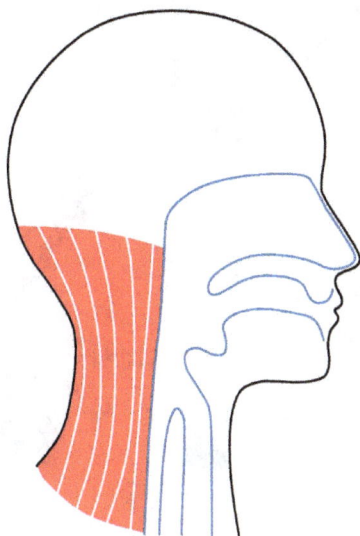

is on the receiving end of their radiated disturbance is thrown into inflammatory chaos!

In the first of these three diagrams, all systems are normal. Blood flow through the neck muscles is uninterrupted with a total absence of pressure point activity or referral.

This second image includes the early signs of stress- and anxiety-related muscular tension and compaction. As you can see, this disturbance (represented by the blackened areas), although relatively minor, has already reduced blood flow and initiated a low-level, generalized reaction (represented by the red-dotted areas) in the remote locations. At this level, still able to function relatively normally, we experience mild indications that all is not well. Things like a fuzzy head, slightly stuffy nose, throat tickle, mildly itchy ear canal, and our eyes don't feel 100 percent. At this moderately increased level of referral activity, our respiratory passages are also more likely to react to airborne irritants.

Lower surface temperatures and increased tension in this third image further clamps the already circulation-compromised neck tissues, amplifying pressure point activity and referral disturbances.

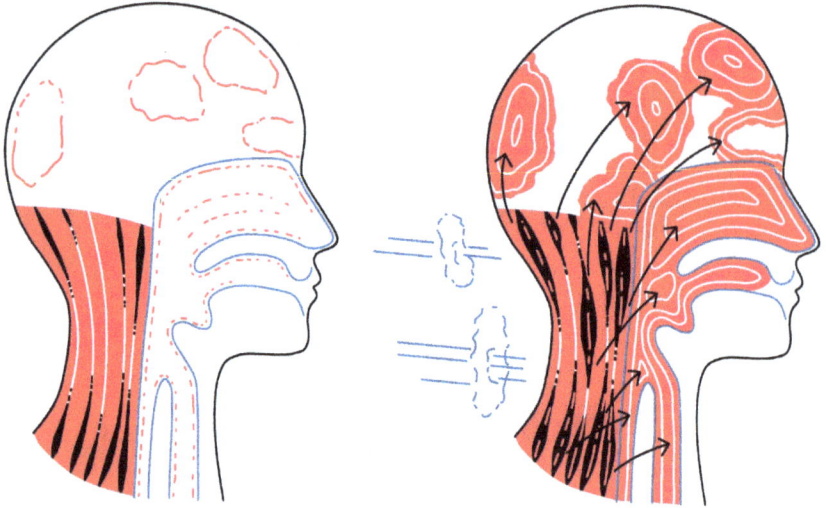

## MARY'S EXPERIENCE

*Symptoms? Red, runny eyes, sore throat, repetitive dry cough, general-ized constant headache, inflamed sinus, and visibly swollen neck glands. A total sceptic, Mary was always relieved to be feeling better after each thirty-minute session and more than a little bemused by how I could clear all of her symptoms by "simply rubbing the back of her neck when hay fever was actually the problem." Mary had become well-versed in "what set it all off this time." Dust, pollen, atmospheric anomalies, smoke, certain foods or drinks, air conditioning . . . The list was familiar and extending. After a decade of intermittent treatments, the one thing con-sistently missing from her triggers list was stress- and anxiety-related tension. You see, all I ever did was gently remobilize Mary's clenched neck. Wearing extra layers helps to prevent us from getting a cold by keeping the tissue containing these pressure points warm, supple, and hydrated. But by far the best protection is to do neck stretches every day.*

# CONCLUSION

This may sound a little strange, but if I could pass just one message to you from this book, it would be to suggest that you feel what happens when you sit on one of your hands. Once your hand has gone through the stages of feeling squashed and a bit painful, it will go numb. This numbness reflects a body whose mind is visiting or living in the stress-filled, anxiety-fuelled life of the red zone. Take a look at your squashed hand and you will see that the blood has been forced out and the tissue has become distorted. This example accurately reflects what happens to our bodies once the mind becomes separated. Once our mind stops listening and responding to our personal alarm system called body pain, we are in trouble. Any brain that decides that it knows better and heads off to do things on its own, independently from the body, will manifest dis-ease. Once you decide to take a few anti-inflammatories and painkillers to continue your isolated, pressured lifestyle, your body will gradually deteriorate. If allowed to continue, this *lifestyle* will eventually stop you. Through chronic illness or dis-ease, you will find yourself removed from your workplace or from society in general. If this does happen and you are lucky enough for your situation not to be terminal, you have a huge task in front of you to *repair the damage that you have done.* In order for a person to make changes, the price of change has to be less than the price of staying the same. For too many of us, our bodies have to actually stop us completely to gain our undivided attention. This, of course, means that if your health suddenly becomes a bigger problem than those you face on a daily basis, you will suddenly have the motivation to do something different. There is an old saying: "*When the student is ready to learn the teacher appears,*" which I think sums up this situation. I have heard so many clients say, "I will do anything to make this pain stop." This is the point of change. At this pivotal point in life, we suddenly realize that we can't trade our body in. We can't swap it for another. This sudden realization can turn us around. And the solution could not be simpler. Listen to your body's alarms and respond appropriately. Sit still every day, even if you can only manage ten or fifteen minutes. Simply stop. Your body never tells lies and will always tell you what it needs. It never stops doing this. All we need to do is listen.

The repair job will not happen overnight. Each of us needs to train ourselves to let go of expecting instant gratification. The road to recovery is usually a long one, but there is no shortcut to anywhere worth being. I suggest that if you are in this situation, start small. Pick one thing to change. Maybe it's drinking a glass of water each day. Or going for a walk, or eating something healthy, or deciding to stop eating something that will foul your body. By picking one thing only and doing it every day for about two months, you initiate a new habit. Once your new habit becomes a part of your everyday life, you won't have to remind yourself to do it. This new healthy habit will then become locked in.

I know the temptation is to add a host of other things, but don't do that. Pick just one more thing to change and do it for the next two months. Alongside these improvements that you can incorporate manually into your life, you will also need to make changes in your thinking and behaviors. If you do what you've always done, you will get what you've always got. So, just like eliminating the weeds from a garden, you're thinking has to bring you away from any thoughts that are powerless and negative. These habitual repetitive thinking patterns can be changed in the same way as we manually increase our exercise, change the foods we eat, and drink more water. You can begin by learning to subtly change a thought, or even a feeling. Catch any thought or feeling and modify it. In the beginning, it doesn't matter whether you make it a bit better or even worse. Tweaking it a tiny wee bit in either direction proves to you that you do have power over how you think and how you feel. Some people like to use positive affirmations, and a simple way to remember to do these is to connect them to something that you already do every day. For example, if you have a mirror in front of you and you've just washed your hands, look into your eyes and take what I call a verbal pill. The verbal pill is a concise repetitive phrase about yourself and your life in a positive vain. Collectively, the changes that you make, however small, begin to wear a new health-enhancing track in your life. These self-help activities of the mind and body replace the negatives on your thought-processing home screen, making them easier to repeat. Another thing that you will notice when you elevate your thinking is that your circle of friends will probably shift. Those people who you are closest to, who insist on continuing to live a dis-eased lifestyle, will gradually disappear from your life. You will naturally begin spending more time with people who resonate with your new self-enhancing way of being. Once you notice this happening, you are well on your way to recovery.

If each of us becomes the best version of ourselves that we possibly can, this will eventually change the world. Once we learn to be kind to ourselves by default, we will start being kind to others. Why? Because we are more likely to share what we have. Once we become comfortable with the truth about ourselves, we become more comfortable being truthful to others. Once we learn to stop harming ourselves, we also learn not to do any harm to others. Once we all learn to slow down our stressful way of living, our society will slow down, because *we* are the ones who are driving the world and everyone in it into destruction. The solution to the problems that our world currently faces, although huge, can be found collectively inside each one of us. You are not your brain. Once you meet resistance from your brain, which has been accustomed to running things, you will know that what you are doing is working. This head resistance appears when you decide to tune in and listen to the center of yourself. Simply sit still and focus on your breathing. As you climb down your seventh-sense virtual ladder from your head into your body, you will begin to discover your true self. This ramps your stress response down to where you can see, hear, feel, smell, and taste fully.

> *Parachutes and minds work a lot better when they are open.*
> *By letting go of your mindsets you could get a lot more than your back back.*

# ACKNOWLEDGMENTS

My Partner Adrienne

Thank you so very much Adrienne for working tirelessly behind the scenes, providing the platform for my work, both in clinic and as I write.

Dr. Joe Brownlee, MBCHB, MRNZCGP, DIP, MSM (Otago)

Deceased 07/10/2022

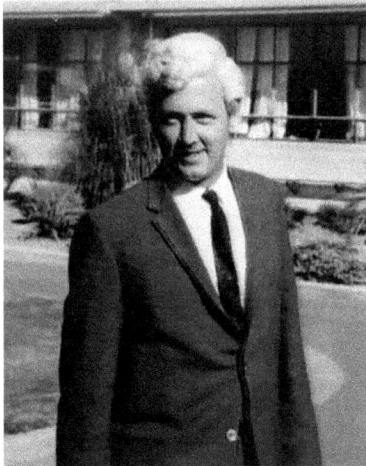

Thank you, Dr. Joe, for your patience, wisdom, and generosity. You tirelessly repeated instructions, ensuring your knowledge was relayed, understood, and reproduced correctly. A truly kind man.

Thanks also to Dr. Stefan N Rheiderer, D.C, MT Chiroprator, and his wife, Corin, who believed in me long before I did, giving me my first real job in the industry.

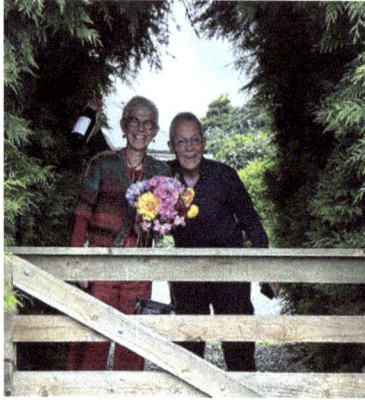

# NOTES

## INTRODUCTION

1. R. A. Hinde and T.E. Rowell, Gestural Communication in Macaques, https://primate.uchicago.edu

2. Susan Jeffers, *Feel the Fear and Do It Anyway*, https://susanjeffers.com

## CHAPTER 4: BACK PAIN USUALLY STARTS IN THE FRONT

1. Roy J. Britten, "Divergence between Samples of Chimpanzee and Human DNA Sequences Is 5%, Counting Indels," *Proc Natl Acad Sci USA*. 2002 Oct 15;99(21):13633-5. doi: 10.1073/pnas.172510699. Epub 2002 Oct 4. PMID: 12368483; PMCID: PMC129726, https://pmc.ncbi.nlm.nih.gov/articles/PMC129726/.

2. "Can Adrenaline Really Lead to Superhuman Strength in Car Accidents?" Gillette Law, P.A., April 8, 2016, https://www.gillettelaw.com/can-adrenaline-really-lead-to-superhuman-strength-in-car-accidents/.

## CHAPTER 5: DISEASE: A STATE OF UNREST

1. Women's Refuge Center Statistic, https://womensrefuge.org.nz.

2. Stress Response Discovery, https://www.scribd.com/document/581500999/Hans-Selye-MD-Wp.

3. Gross Body Movement Citation, https://pmc.ncbi.nim.nih.gov.

4. Medino Online, https://www.medino.com.

5. W Cancer Deaths, https://www.who.int.

## CHAPTER 6: REINVIGORATION

1. Dr. Michael Mosley, https://.bbc.uk.

   You Tube, "Can You Change Your Body in Three Weeks?"

## CHAPTER 7: BORN BEHIND THE EIGHT BALL

1. Rob Levy, "Remembrance of Things Past: Adult Cells Maintain Complete Molecular 'Memory' of Their Embryonic Origins," Harvard Medical School, March 21, 2019, https://hms.harvard.edu/news/remembrance-things-past.

2. Bill Bryson, *Short History of Nearly Everything* (Crown, 2003).

## CHAPTER 8: LIFE ABOVE THE RED LINE

1. Noa Kegamaya PhD, Worry, https://bulletproofmusician.com.

2. Sandy Loder, "The Impact of 45,000 Negative Thoughts," Peak Dynamics, March 10, 2023, https://insights.peak-dynamics.net/post/102ia4i/the-impact-of-45-000-negative-thoughts.

3. Jay Summer and Dr. Pranshu Adavadkar, "What Is a NASA Nap? How to Power Naplike an Astronaut," Sleep Foundation, October 27, 2023, https://www.sleepfoundation.org/sleep-hygiene/nasa-nap#:~:text=The%20original%201995%20NASA%20study,those%20who%20didn't%20nap.

4. Martin Luther quote, Goodreads, Inc., https://www.goodreads.com/work/quotes/531939-von-der-freiheit-eines-christenmenschen.

## CHAPTER 11: BREATH OR DEATH

1. Queen of the Desert, https://youtu.be/nljWBU2hF_A?si=oj6hWs1ZvgVYz97l.

## CHAPTER 13: STRESS-RELATED HOLDING PATTERNS

1. National Institute of Health, https://pubmed.ncbinlm.nih.gov.

## CHAPTER 18: FOOD FOR THOUGHT

1. Rachel Hunter, *Rachel Hunter's Tour of Beauty* (Affirm Press, 2020).

2. John Steinbeck, *The Grapes of Wrath* (The Viking Press, 1939).

3. Marcue E. Raichle and Debrah A. Gusnard, "Appraising the Brain's Energy Budget," *Proc Natl Acad Sci USA*. 2002 Aug 6;99(16):10237-9. doi: 10.1073/

pnas.172399499. Epub 2002 Jul 29. PMID: 12149485; PMCID: PMC124895.https://
pmc.ncbi.nlm.nih.gov/articles/PMC124895/.

4. Alone TV Series, https://www.netflix.com/title/81271131.

   https://www.amazon.com/Alone-Season-1/dp/B00ZOSJOLY.

5. Janet G. Travell, MD and David G. Simons, *The Trigger Point Manual*
   (Lippincott Williams & Wilkins, 1994).

# ABOUT THE AUTHOR

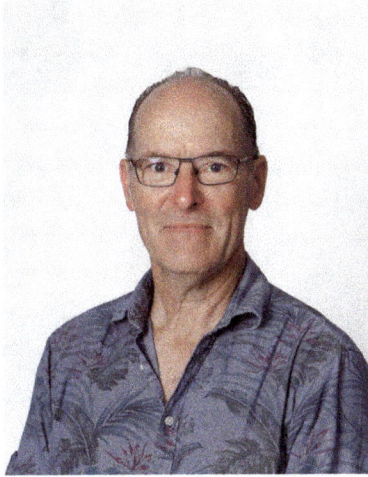

Alistair Fergus McKenzie an advanced trade electrician for twenty-five years specializing in the installation and maintenance of solar and diesel-electric power supplies, whose hobby of healing others transitioned into professional therapeutic massage following his certification in 2001. Three years of part-time clinical training in musculoskeletal technique saw his practice evolve into manual therapy, which he still does three days weekly, although he has been "retired" for three years. Redirecting his innate curiosity and natural fault/cause finding ability to repair things electromechanical toward the dysfunctions of the human body, Alistair has unraveled some of the mystery surrounding mind-body connections. He currently lives in New Zealand with his partner, Adrienne.

www.ingramcontent.com/pod-product-compliance
Lightning Source LLC
Chambersburg PA
CBHW070608270326
41926CB00013B/2468